Obs and Gynae

PG Focus Series

Pyrexia in Pregnancy

Obs and Gynae
PG Focus Series
Pyrexia in Pregnancy

Editors

Komal N Chavan

MD DNB MNAMS FCPS DGO FICOG and Diploma in Reproductive Medicine (UK-SH Germany)

Senior Consultant and Unit Chief

Department of Obstetrics and Gynaecology

VN Desai Hospital

Mumbai, Maharashtra, India

Niranjan Chavan

MD FICOG FCPS DGO DFP MICOG DICOG Diploma in Endoscopy (USA)

Professor and Unit Chief

Department of Obstetrics and Gynaecology

Lokmanya Tilak Medical College and General Hospital

Mumbai, Maharashtra, India

Co-Editors

Akanksha Barkase

MBBS MS (Obs/Gynae) DNB FMAS

Consultant Obstetrician and Gynaecologist

Department of Obstetrics and Gynaecology

Kaushalya Hospital

Dhule, Maharashtra, India

Shikhanshi

MBBS MS DNB (Obs/Gynae)

Assisted Professor

Department of Obstetrics and Gynaecology

Topiwala National Medical College and BYL Nair Charitable Hospital

Mumbai, Maharashtra, India

JAYPEE

JAYPEE BROTHERS MEDICAL PUBLISHERS

The Health Sciences Publisher

New Delhi | London

Jaypee Brothers Medical Publishers (P) Ltd

Headquarters
Jaypee Brothers Medical Publishers (P) Ltd
EMCA House, 23/23-B
Ansari Road, Daryaganj
New Delhi 110 002, India
Landline: +91-11-23272143, +91-11-23272703
+91-11-23282021, +91-11-23245672
Email: jaypee@jaypeebrothers.com

Corporate Office
Jaypee Brothers Medical Publishers (P) Ltd
4838/24, Ansari Road, Daryaganj
New Delhi 110 002, India
Phone: +91-11-43574357
Fax: +91-11-43574314
Email: jaypee@jaypeebrothers.com

Overseas Office
JP Medical Ltd.
83, Victoria Street, London
SW1H 0HW (UK)
Phone: +44 20 3170 8910
Fax: +44 (0)20 3008 6180
Email: info@jpmedpub.com

Website: www.jaypeebrothers.com
Website: www.jaypeedigital.com

Inquiries for bulk sales may be solicited at: jaypee@jaypeebrothers.com

Obs and Gynae PG Focus Series: Pyrexia in Pregnancy

First Edition: **2025**

ISBN: 978-93-6616-843-2

Printed in India

Preface

Fever in pregnancy can have far-reaching implications for both mother and fetus, increasing the risk of complications, preterm labor, and even birth defects. Despite its significance, pyrexia in pregnancy remains a topic of ongoing debate and discussion among healthcare professionals.

This book aims to provide a comprehensive and authoritative guide to *Pyrexia in Pregnancy*, drawing on the latest research, clinical guidelines, and expert opinions. This book is written for healthcare providers, researchers, and pregnant individuals alike and seeks to illuminate the complexities of pyrexia in pregnancy while offering practical insights and evidence-based strategies for management and care.

Through this book, we hope to contribute meaningfully to the existing body of knowledge on pyrexia in pregnancy, ultimately enhancing maternal and fetal outcomes and improving the quality-of-care for pregnant individuals worldwide.

Editors
Komal N Chavan
Niranjan Chavan

Co-Editors
Akanksha Barkase
Shikhanshi

Acknowledgments

We express our heartfelt gratitude to everyone who contributed to the completion of this book, *Pyrexia in Pregnancy*. This endeavor would not have been possible without the invaluable support and encouragement of many individuals.

We sincerely thank all the Authors and Co-authors for their dedication and expertise in creating a resource of the highest academic and clinical standards.

Our gratitude extends to our mentors and colleagues for their insightful guidance and constructive feedback, which shaped the structure and content of this book.

We are deeply thankful to our families and friends for their steadfast support, patience, and encouragement during the challenging phases of this project. Their unwavering belief in us has been a constant source of strength and inspiration.

We acknowledge the invaluable support of Shri Jitendar P Vij (Group Chairman) and Mr Ankit Vij (Managing Director) of M/s Jaypee Brothers Medical Publishers (P) Ltd, New Delhi, India, for their pivotal role in bringing this book to fruition. We extend special thanks to their team, particularly Ms Chetna Malhotra (Senior Director—Professional Publishing, Marketing, and Business Development), Ms Kritika Dua (Senior Commissioning Editor), Ms Pragati Singh, and Mr Priyansh Saxena (Development Editors), for their professionalism, efficiency, and consistent assistance throughout the publishing process.

We hope this book serves as a valuable resource in enhancing patient care and clinical outcomes, as well as a comprehensive and practical guide for postgraduate students, helping them excel in their examinations. Finally, we aim for it to serve as a quick-reference tool for teachers and practicing FOGSIans.

Thank you all for being an integral part of this journey.

Contents

1 CHAPTER Introduction

Fever, also known as pyrexia, is a condition in which the body's temperature rises above its normal range due to an increase in the body's temperature set point, which is usually greater than 37.7°C or 99.9°F.

The hypothalamus regulates body temperature. Neurons in the preoptic anterior hypothalamus and posterior hypothalamus get two types of signals: one from peripheral nerves transmitting information from skin warmth/cold receptors, and the other from the temperature of the blood soaking the region.

To maintain normal temperatures, the thermoregulatory center of the hypothalamus integrates these two types of signals. The human metabolic rate produces more heat than is required to keep the core body temperature between 36.5 and 37.5°C (97.7 and 99.5°F) in a neutral temperature environment.

The average daily temperature variation, often known as the circadian rhythm, is 0.5°C.

The temperature of women in the reproductive age group is normally lower during the 2 weeks preceding ovulation, rises by 0.6°C with ovulation, and remains at that level until menses occur. The amplitude of the circadian rhythm remains constant during the luteal phase.

PATHOGENESIS OF FEVER

Pyrogens: Greek for fire, is used to describe any substance that causes fever. It may be classified as exogenous or endogenous.

Pyrogenic cytokines: Cytokines causing fever are called pyrogenic cytokines and include interleukin-1 (IL-1), IL-6, tumor necrosis factor (TNF), and ciliary neurotropic factor.

The hypothalamic set point increases, causing peripheral vasoconstriction. As a result of blood shunting to the internal organs, the patient feels cold. Shivering and enhanced hepatic thermogenesis are examples of heat-producing mechanisms that aid in raising the body temperature to the new set point. The nonspecific myalgia and arthralgia that frequently accompany fever are due to an increase in peripheral prostaglandin E2. When the set point is decreased again due to the resolution or treatment of a fever, heat loss mechanisms begin (e.g., peripheral vasodilatation and sweating) commence.

Figure 1 highlights the pathogenesis pathway of fever.

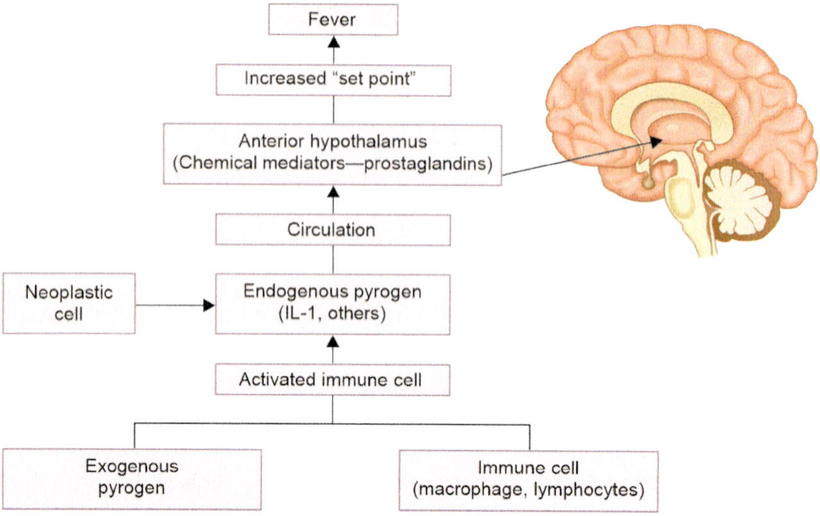

Fig. 1: Pathway of development of fever.
Source: Adapted from Miller JB. Hyperthermia and fever of unknown origin. In: Ettinger SJ, Feldman EC (Eds). Textbook of veterinary internal medicine, 6th edition. St Louis: Saunders; 2005.

SUGGESTED READING

1. Jameson J. Harrison's principles of internal medicine, 20th edition. New York, NY: McGraw-Hill Education; 2018.
2. Williams J, Cunningham F, Levenovo K, Bloom S, Hauth J, Gilstrap L, et al. Obstetrics, 25th edition. Estados Unidos: McGraw-Hill; 2005.

2

CHAPTER

Approach to a Pregnant Patient with Fever

INTRODUCTION

The approach to a patient with fever should include a comprehensive history, clinical examination, appropriate lab investigations which will aid in finding out the cause of fever.

HISTORY

A thorough history is required, with special attention paid to the sequence of events (for example, in the case of a rash, the site of onset as well as the direction and rate of spread) and the relationship of symptoms to medications, previous exposure, sick contacts, sexual contacts, travel, trauma, and the presence of prosthetic materials.

PHYSICAL EXAMINATION

A thorough physical examination is most necessary part. Temperature should be taken from one particular point. Temperature and pulse association should be noted. The weeks of pregnancy and the onset of symptoms at which age of gestation should be noted which will guide the treatment required and history of similar symptoms in antecedent pregnancy. Any history of urinary complaints or leaking/bleeding per vaginum should require a per speculum examination.

Close attention should be given to the presence of any rash, with precise definition of its salient feature.

- *Lesion type:* Macule, papule, nodule, vesicle, pustule, purpura, and ulcer
- *Configuration:* Annular or target
- *Arrangement and distribution:* Central or peripheral

Types of rashes:

- *Central eruptions mainly maculopapular:* Viral exanthems, exanthematous drug-induced eruptions
- *Peripheral eruptions:* Rocky Mountain spotted fever, secondary syphilis, bacterial endocarditis
- *Confluent desquamative erythemas:* Toxic shock syndrome
- *Vesiculobullous eruption:* Varicella, primary HSV infection, ecthyma gangrenosum

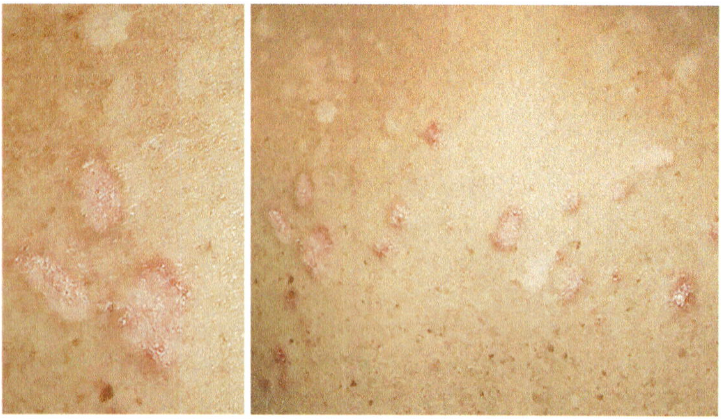

Fig. 1: Rash in a female having autoimmune disease.

- *Urticaria like eruptions:* Serum sickness, connective tissue disorder, viral infections, malignancy like lymphoma
- *Nodular eruption:* Disseminated fungal infection, erythema nodosum, sweet syndrome
- *Purpuric eruptions:* Meningococcemia, viral hemorrhagic fever, disseminated gonococcemia
- Autoimmune disorders **(Fig. 1)**

LABORATORY TESTS

Basic investigations that should be sent in a patient complaining of fever are:

- Complete blood count
- Erythrocyte sedimentation rate (ESR)
- C-reactive protein
- Urine routine microscopy
- Peripheral blood smear for parasites
- Dengue and Leptospira Ag
- High vaginal swab

TREATMENT

Antipyretics are not contraindicated in pregnancy and can be given in viral and bacterial infections without slowing the resolution of infection. In cases where diagnosis of fever is to be made by pattern of fever and its association with pulse, withholding of antipyretic may be required.

Aspirin, nonsteroidal anti-inflammatory drugs (NSAIDs), and glucocorticoids are effective antipyretics. However, NSAIDs should not be used beyond 28 weeks as it may cause premature closure of ductus arteriosus. Acetaminophen is preferable since it does not promote inflammation, does not decrease platelet function, and does not cause Reye's syndrome. In addition to oral antipyretics, hyperpyretic patients should be treated with cooling blankets. Strict monitoring of fetal heart rate and daily fetal kick counts should be done.

CONCLUSION

It is important to note significant clinical findings and order necessary investigations. Antipyretics are the first line treatment for fever in pregnancy. Care must be taken with use of NSAIDs beyond 28 weeks.

SUGGESTED READING

1. Jameson J. Harrison's principles of internal medicine, 20th edition. New York, NY: McGraw-Hill Education; 2018.
2. Williams J, Cunningham F, Leveno K, Bloom S, Hauth J, Gilstrap L, et al. Obstetrics, 25th edition. Estados Unidos: McGraw-Hill; 2005.

3

CHAPTER

Infectious Causes of Pyrexia in Pregnancy

Systemic Causes

INTRODUCTION

Causes of fever may be classified depending upon location of infection or the causative organism.

For further study, we will divide infection into:

- Systematic causes
- Local causes

Systematic causes can be further divided according to cause into:

- Bacterial
- Viral
- Parasitic infections

Local causes which are specific to pregnancy may be divided into:

- Intra-amniotic infection
- Genital infection/vaginal infection
- Urinary tract infection
- Skin and soft tissue infection

BACTERIAL INFECTIONS IN PREGNANCY

TUBERCULOSIS

Tuberculosis (TB) is caused by *Mycobacterium tuberculosis* which is an acid-fast bacillus. TB bacteria are most commonly found in the lungs, although they can also be found in the kidney, spine, and brain. Not everyone, who is infected with the tuberculosis bacteria, becomes ill. As a result, there are two TB-related conditions: Latent tuberculosis infection (LTBI) and tuberculosis illness. TB disease can be lethal if not treated appropriately. TB is a bacterial infection spread through inhaling tiny droplets from the coughs or sneezes of an infected person. In early times, when treatment of TB was not present, it was considered a death sentence.

Typical symptoms of TB include:

- A persistent cough that lasts >3 weeks and is usually associated with expectoration and may be associated with hemoptysis

- Weight loss
- Night sweats
- High temperature
- Tiredness and fatigue
- Loss of appetite
- Swellings in the neck

Systems Involved

Tuberculosis mostly effects the pulmonary system but may include—renal, intestinal, and skeletal TB.

Tubercular meningitis is most fatal and may mimic hyperemesis gravidarum in early stages. Spinal tuberculosis may cause paraplegia and may also cause bone deformity and psoas abscess. Extrapulmonary tuberculosis usually has late diagnosis.

Effects on Pregnancy

Effects on pregnancy usually depend on gestational age and diagnosis. Active untreated pulmonary infections can cause:

- Preterm delivery
- Low birth weight
- Growth restriction
- Preeclampsia
- Perinatal mortality

Diagnosis

Following tests may be used for diagnosis of tuberculosis:

- Chest X-ray posteroanterior (PA) view with abdominal shield to test the severity of pulmonary TB **(Fig. 1)**
- Sputum/fluid acid-fast bacilli staining **(Fig. 2)**
- Sputum/fluid Löwenstein-Jensen (LJ) media culture sensitivity
- Ascitic/pleural fluid ADA levels
- Tuberculin skin test (not valid if BCG vaccine taken)
- Interferon gamma release assay (*QuantiFERON-TB Gold* and *T-SPOT TB*)
- *Xpert MTB/RIF commercially* available diagnostic test that uses polymerase chain reaction (PCR)

Treatment

For new TB cases, the treatment in:

- *Intensive phase (IP):* Isoniazid (INH), rifampicin, pyrazinamide, and ethambutol (HRZE) in daily doses for 8 weeks
- *Continuation phase (CP):* Three drug FDCs—rifampicin, isoniazid, and ethambutol (HRE) are continued for 16 weeks.

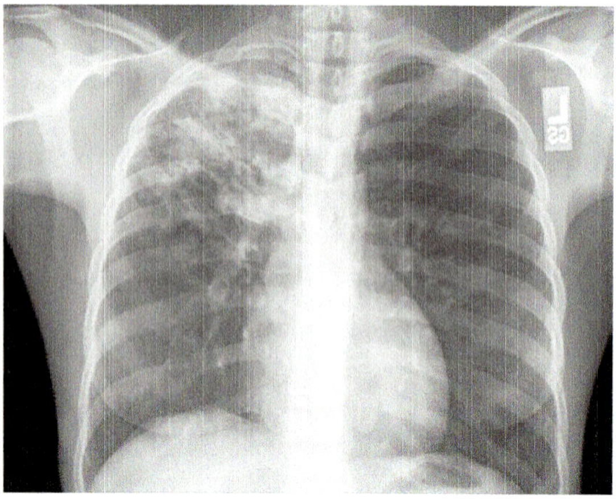

Fig. 1: Chest X-ray PA view of a person affected with TB. (PA: posteroanterior; TB: tuberculosis)
Source: Gaillard F. Pulmonary tuberculosis. Case study. [online] Available from https://radiopaedia.org/cases/8632. [Last accessed November, 2024]

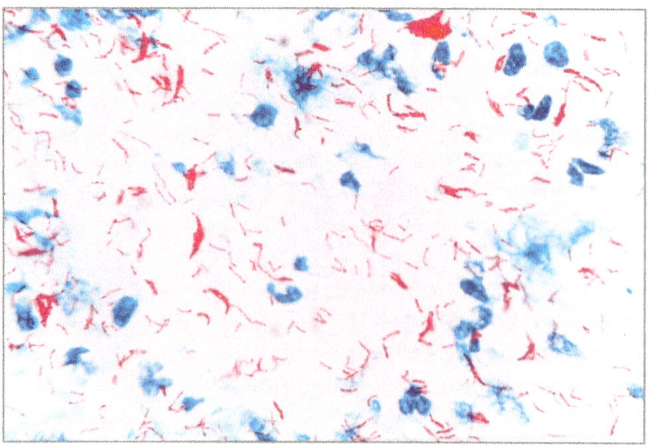

Fig. 2: *Mycobacterium tuberculosis* on acid-fast stain.
Source: The Rockefeller University. (2018). Study identifies genetic mutation responsible for tuberculosis vulnerability. [online] Available from https://www.rockefeller.edu/news/24686-study-identifies-genetic-mutation-responsible-tuberculosis-vulnerability. [Last accessed November, 2024]

Pregnant and breastfeeding women may be treated with RHZE, i.e., rifampicin, isoniazid, pyrazinamide, and ethambutol with pyridoxine 10 mg daily, as for other patients. There is no need to cease breastfeeding.

For previously treated cases of TB:

- *Intensive phase* constitutes of 12 weeks, in which injectable drug—streptomycin is given for 8 weeks along with four drugs (isoniazid, rifampicin, pyrazinamide, and ethambutol) and after 8 weeks the four drugs (isoniazid, rifampicin, pyrazinamide, and ethambutol) in daily doses as per weight bands are continued for another 4 weeks

- *Continuation phase:* Rifampicin, isoniazid, and ethambutol are continued for next 20 weeks daily.

Some drugs used in secondary regimens such as streptomycin, protionamide, ethionamide, and the quinolones are contraindicated due to teratogenicity.

In TB meningitis or pericarditis, addition of corticosteroids in HIV-negative females is beneficial.

Neonatal Tuberculosis

Neonates can be infected by two ways, either through placenta (congenital tuberculosis) or by aspiration of secretions at time of delivery.

Symptoms include:

- Hepatosplenomegaly
- Respiratory distress
- Fever
- Lymphadenopathy

Chances of infection decrease if the mother with active disease has been treated before delivery or her sputum culture report is negative. If untreated, the risk of infection to newborn in 1st year is as high as 50% and isolation from mother is required.

TYPHOID FEVER

Infection from typhoid fever is a major cause of food-borne diseases. It is gram-negative bacilli of *Enterobacteriaceae* family. Most common subtypes found in India causing typhoid fever are *Salmonella typhi* and *Salmonella paratyphi.*

Susceptibility is increased by conditions that diminish gastric acidity or intestinal integrity.

Organisms pass through the mucus layers of the small intestine and into the intestinal epithelium via M cells covering Peyer's patches.

Incubation period of 5–21 days. It is a systemic disease.

Signs and symptoms include:

- Fever which may be prolonged
- Abdominal pain
- Anorexia
- Headache
- Chills
- Sweating
- Diarrhea

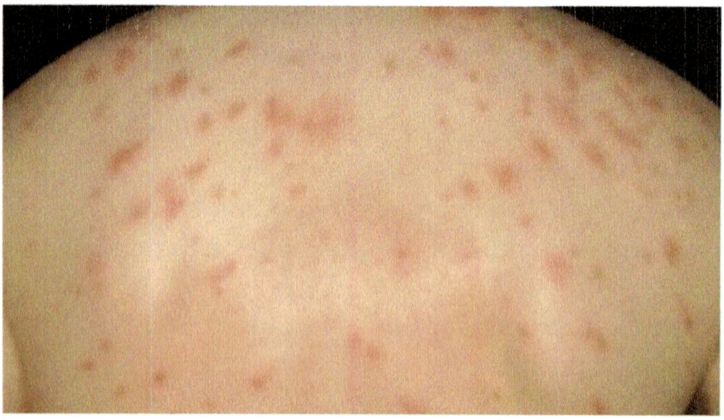

Fig. 3: Rose spots seen in typhoid.
Source: McConnell A. (2020). Fever, Abdominal pain, Constipation and Mary. [online] Available from https://litfl.com/fever-abdominal-pain-constipation-and-mary/. [Last accessed November, 2024]

- Less often constipation
- Rose spots **(Fig. 3)**
- Relative bradycardia
- Hepatosplenomegaly

Long-term *Salmonella* carriers develop in 1–5% cases.

Nontyphoidal salmonellosis is caused by *S. typhimurium or S. enteritidis* acquired mainly from animal reservoirs.

Effects on Pregnancy

Antepartum typhoid infection can cause:
- Abortion
- Preterm labor
- Maternal or fetal death

Diagnosis

Diagnosis can be done by:
- *1st week:* Blood culture
- *2nd week onwards:* Agglutination test (WIDAL)
- *3rd week onwards:* Stool culture
- *4th week onwards:* Urine culture

Isolation on bacilli is the gold standard test. **Figure 4** shows *Salmonella typhi* under microscope. WIDAL is tube agglutination done which is most commonly done. The titer is specific to each population according to the endemicity of bacteria in that region.

Treatment

Fluoroquinolones and third-generation cephalosporins are the preferred treatment.

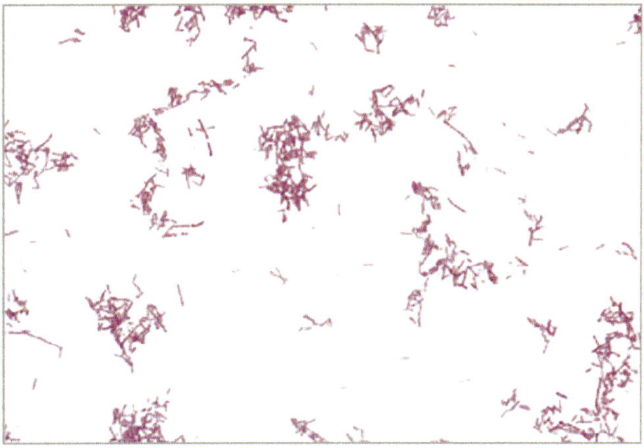

Fig. 4: *Salmonella typhi* under microscope.
Source: Avantor. Salmonella typhimurium Slide. [online] Available from https://pr.vwr.com/store/product/8886425/salmonella-typhimurium-slide. [Last accessed November, 2024]

Intravenous hydration and treatment of dehydration may be required. Dexamethasone may be beneficial in severe cases.

LEPTOSPIROSIS

Humans and animals are both affected by leptospirosis, a bacterial disease. Leptospira is a genus of spirochaete bacteria that includes a small number of pathogenic and saprophytic species (*Ancient Greek:* Leptos, "fine, thin" and *Latin:* Spira, "coil" seen in **Figure 5**). Leptospira was initially discovered in kidney tissue slices of a leptospirosis victim who had died of "yellow fever" in 1907. It can induce a wide range of symptoms in humans, some of which may be misdiagnosed as other illnesses. Some infected people, on the other hand, may show no signs or symptoms at all.

Leptospirosis can cause renal disorders, liver disorders, meningitis, respiratory difficulty, and even death if left untreated.

Epidemiology

The bacteria that cause leptospirosis are disseminated by diseased animals' urine, which can enter water or soil and live for weeks to months. The bacteria are carried by a wide range of wild and domestic animals. When these animals become sick, they may show no signs of illness.

For a few months to several years, infected animals may continue to discharge bacteria into the environment on a regular or irregular basis.

Humans can become infected in the following ways:

- Contact with infected animals' urine (or other body fluids, except saliva)
- Contact with diseased animals' urine contaminated water, food, or soil

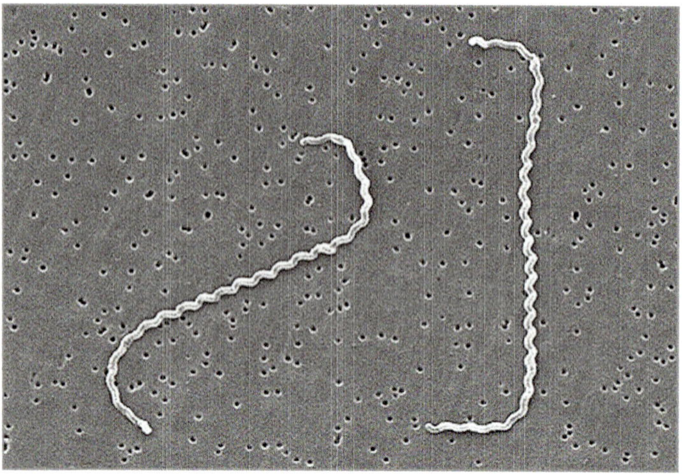

Fig. 5: Microscopic appearance of leptospirosis.
Source: Wikipedia. Leptospira. [online] Available from https://www.google.com/url?sa=i&url=https%3A%2F%2Fen.wikipedia.org%2Fwiki%2FLeptospira&psig=AOvVaw1sp4_n69SuZZKLrZbBnpfT&ust=1644332446219000& source=images&cd=vfe&ved=0CAsQjRxqFwoTCJiEkfLt7fUCFQAAAAAdAAAAABAD. [Last accessed November, 2024]

The bacteria enter the body through the skin or mucous membranes (eyes, nose, and mouth), particularly if the skin has any abrasion or loss of integrity. Infection can also be spread by drinking polluted water. Leptospirosis outbreaks are usually induced by contact with polluted water, such as flooding. Transmission from one person to another is uncommon.

Clinical Features

Leptospirosis can produce a variety of symptoms in people, including:

- High-grade fever with chills
- Headache
- Myalgia
- Vomiting
- Jaundice
- Pain in the abdomen
- Diarrhea
- Rash

Weil's disease is an acute, severe form of leptospirosis that produces jaundice (yellow skin and eyes), renal failure, and bleeding in the sick person. Severe pulmonary hemorrhage syndrome refers to pulmonary bleeding caused by leptospirosis.

Conjunctival suffusion (red conjunctiva) **(Fig. 6)** together with jaundice is a specific feature of leptospirosis.

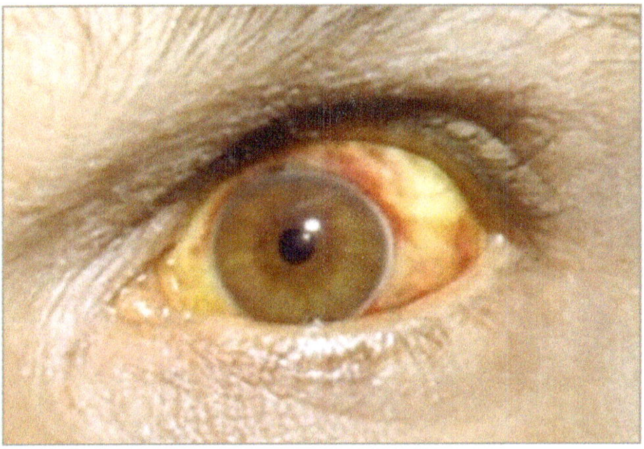

Fig. 6: Conjunctival suffusion.
Source: WikEM. Conjunctivalsuffusion.jpg. [online] Available from https://wikem.org/wiki/File:Conjunctivalsuffusion.jpg#filelinks. [Last accessed November, 2024]

Leptospirosis is endemic in most regions where the dengue virus is spread, and it is sometimes confused with dengue, which is more common. In up to 8% of instances, co-infection occurs.

The incubation period ranges from 2 to 4 weeks. Fever and other symptoms are frequently the first signs of illness.

Leptospirosis can be divided into two stages:
1. *First phase:* Fever, chills, headache, muscle aches, vomiting, or diarrhea
2. *Second phase:* Renal failure, liver failure, meningitis

The disease might persist anywhere from a few days to 3 weeks or more.

Leptospirosis can be found all throughout the world; however, it is most frequent in temperate and tropical areas. It is an occupational danger for many persons who work with animals or in the outdoors, such as:
- Farmers
- Mine employees
- Workers in the sewers
- Those who work at slaughterhouses are known as "slaughterhouse laborers."
- Animal carers and veterinarians
- Employees who deal with fish
- Farmers that produce milk
- Personnel from the military

Leptospirosis is an amalgamation of factors involving the host, environment, and pathogen. **Figure 7** further explains this triad.

Swimming, wading, kayaking, and rafting in contaminated lakes and rivers have also been linked to the disease. As a result, campers and outdoor

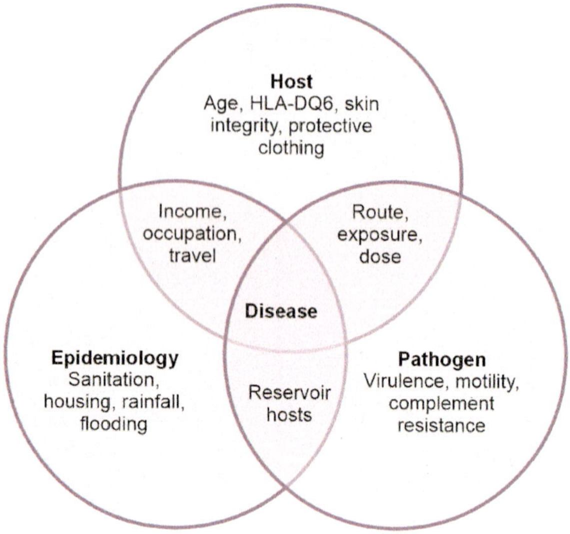

Fig. 7: The triad of disease leptospirosis.
Source: Haake DA, Levett PN. (2015). Leptospirosis in humans. [online] Available from https://www.ncbi.nlm.nih.gov/pmc/articles/PMC4442676/. [Last accessed November, 2024]

sports lovers face a recreational hazard. Those who engage in these activities in tropical or temperate regions are more likely to be at danger.

Furthermore, the prevalence of leptospirosis infection in urban youngsters appears to be rising.

In pregnancy, the disease has shown to cause acute maternal illness leading to intrauterine growth restriction (IUGR), preterm delivery, and even intrauterine fetal death (IUFD). The disease can initially be confused with HELLP, AFLP, cholestasis of pregnancy, or idiopathic thrombocytopenia of pregnancy. Thus, early suspicion is very essential in cases of fever to improve maternal and fetal outcome.

Diagnosis

Laboratory diagnosis is crucial because of the nonspecific clinical presentation; however, typical diagnostic methods are so slow and occasionally imprecise that they are of limited help when they are most needed.

Blood and urine cultures taken during the feverish period (1st 7–10 days of disease, not of hospitalization) are helpful and come positive, but bacteria grow slowly and may not show up in standard laboratory tests for 2–3 weeks or more.

Meanwhile, treatment must be started right away if a presumptive diagnosis is made. Although molecular (PCR-based) approaches are more sensitive and faster than culture, probes are not uniformly suitable to all serovars.

As a result, serological tests are still used to make diagnoses.

The most specific and precise test is the microscopic agglutination test (MAT).

A positive reaction is defined as a titer of 1:400-1:800 or higher in a single test, or a rising titer to these levels in paired sera over the first 2 or 3 weeks; a positive reaction is defined as a titer of 1:400–1:800 or higher in a single test, or a titer which is rising up to these levels in paired sera over the first 2 or 3 weeks.

The maximum serum titer varies by serovar; however, it is usually reached after 3–4 weeks of sickness.

It gradually fades after that. Because a clear positive result is a direct guide to diagnosis, treatment, and management, the initial serum sample should be analyzed without waiting for the second of a pair.

Treatment

Intravenous penicillin (1.5 million units IV every 6 hours), ampicillin (0.5–1 g IV every 6 hours), ceftriaxone (1 g IV every 24 hours), or cefotaxime are commonly used for patients with severe leptospirosis who require hospitalization (1 g IV every 6 h).

Ceftriaxone has been demonstrated to be noninferior to penicillin in the treatment of serious leptospirosis, and offers the benefit of intramuscular injection as an alternative to intravenous medication in situations when hospitalization is not available.

Adult cases with early illness should take either 100 mg of doxycycline two times daily or 500 mg of azithromycin once daily.

In pregnant females and children: Ampicillin and azithromycin can be given in weight-adjusted dosage.

GROUP A STREPTOCOCCUS

Infections caused by *Streptococcus pyogenes* are important in pregnant women. It may cause:

- Acute pharyngitis
- Severe systemic and cutaneous infections
- Scarlet fever
- Erysipelas/cellulitis
- Necrotizing fasciitis/myositis
- Impetigo
- Pneumonia/empyema
- Streptococcal toxic shock syndrome
- Puerperal sepsis

Streptococcus pyogenes produces numerous toxins and enzymes which cause local and systemic toxicity.

Effects on Pregnancy

- Preterm labor
- Chorioamnionitis
- Sepsis
- Multiorgan failure
- Maternal morbidity
- Fetal morbidity and mortality

Diagnosis

- Gram staining **(Fig. 8)**
- Culture test
- Catalase test

Treatment

Main line of treatment is symptomatic management with beta-lactamase antibiotics.

In skin infection, debridement is required.

- Penicillin G 2–4-million unit IV 4 hourly with clindamycin in severe cases
- Penicillin G 1.2-million unit IM or penicillin V 250 mg TDS for 10 days in less severe cases.
  In cases of penicillin allergy, first-generation cephalosporin can be given.

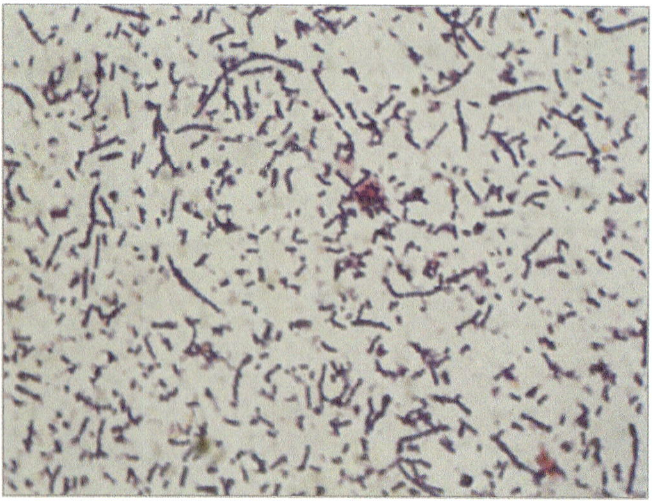

Fig. 8: Group A streptococcus on Gram staining.
Source: Ramana KV, Reddy KM, Palange P, Rao BM, Rao SD. Cerebral Abscess Caused by Streptococcus spp in a Patient with Chronic Suppurative Otitis Media (CSOM). Am J Infect Dis Microbiol. 2014;2(5):131-7.

GROUP B STREPTOCOCCUS

Most group B Streptococcus (GBS) infections in adults are seen in pregnancy and postpartum. *S. agalactiae* is a group B Streptococcus that can be found to colonize in gastrointestinal and genitourinary tract of 10–25% pregnant females.

Effects in Pregnancy

The effects range from asymptomatic colonization to septicemia.

- Preterm labor
- Prematurely ruptured membranes
- Clinical and subclinical chorioamnionitis
- Fetal infections
- Maternal bacteriuria
- Pyelonephritis
- Osteomyelitis
- Postpartum mastitis
- Puerperal infections

Neonatal sepsis is the one of the most devastating sequelae of GBS which is easily preventable.

Diagnosis

Culture is the mainstay of diagnosis.

- High vaginal swab
- Rectal swab
- Urine culture
- Pus culture

Treatment

Penicillin is the first line of treatment. In patients sensitive to penicillin, vancomycin can be used.

Neonatal Infections

Group B streptococcus is the major cause of meningitis and sepsis in neonates. About half of infants delivered vaginally to mothers colonized with GBS become colonized and about 1–2% become infected. The risk of infection increases if there is:

- Preterm delivery
- Early rupture of membranes (>24 hours)
- Prolonged labor
- Fever
- Chorioamnionitis

Figure 9 shows the spectrum of infection of GBS.

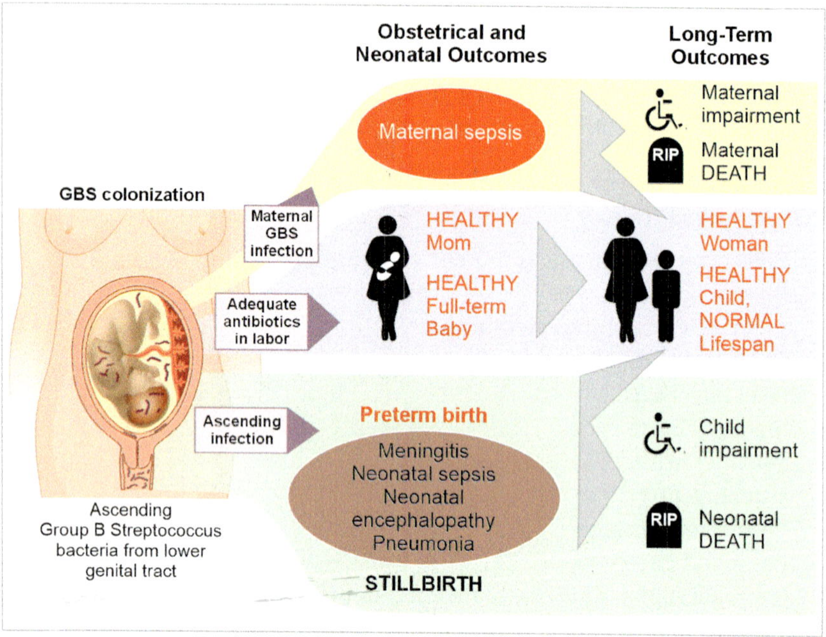

Fig. 9: Group B streptococcus spectrum of infection.
Source: Armistead B, Oler E, Adams Waldorf K, Rajagopal L. The Double Life of Group B Streptococcus: Asymptomatic Colonizer and Potent Pathogen. J Mol Biol. 2019;431(16):2914-31.

Infections can be of two types:

1. *Early onset:* Occurs within 1st week of life. The infection is acquired through maternal genital tract during delivery. Symptoms include respiratory distress, lethargy, and hypotension.

   If symptoms develop <72 hours of life, intrauterine infection is suspected.

   Bacteremia is present in around 100% cases, pneumonia in one-third to half and meningitis in one-third.
2. *Late onset:* Occurs in infants >1 week but <3 months of age. Infection is acquired during delivery or later. Meningitis is the most common manifestation. Symptoms include lethargy, fever, irritability, poor feeding, and may be seizures.

Prophylaxis: It can be done in two approaches, mainly culture-based prevention and risk-based prevention. Intrapartum prophylaxis is indicated in the following cases:

- Previous infant with invasive GBS disease
- GBS bacteriuria in current pregnancy
- Positive GBS culture during current pregnancy

Flowchart 1: Pathway of care for preventing early onset neonatal GBS sepsis.

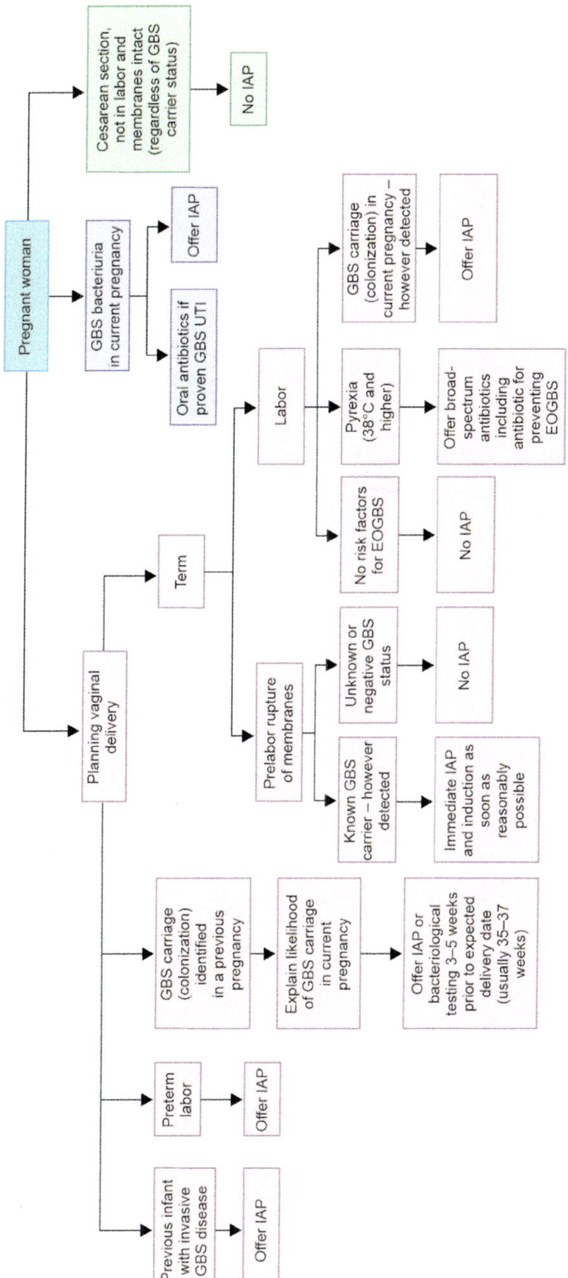

(GBS: group B streptococcus)

- Unknown GBS status with preterm labor
- Premature rupture/prolonged rupture of membranes
- Intrapartum temperature >100.4°F
- Intrapartum nucleic acid amplification test (NAAT) positive for GBS

Penicillin G 5 million units IV loading dose followed by 2.5–3 million units IV every 4 hourly until delivery.

Alternatively, injection ampicillin 2 g IV then 2 g IV every 4 hour till delivery.

Patients allergic to penicillin may receive cephazolin/clindamycin or vancomycin.

Flowchart 1 highlights the pathway of care for women with history of GBS infection and current GBS infection.

VIRAL INFECTIONS IN PREGNANCY

INFLUENZA VIRUS

These viruses generally infect the respiratory tract and belong to the family orthomyxoviridae. They can be divided into influenza A and B viruses. Influenza A viruses can be classified further on the basis of their surface antigens—hemagglutinin (H) and neuraminidase (N). **Figure 10** shows structure of influenza virus. Influenza outbreaks occur annually and may cause epidemic/pandemic. The symptoms generally include:

- Fever
- Cold
- Dry cough

Effects in Pregnancy

Systemic infection is generally nonlife threatening in healthy adults but pregnant females are more susceptible to this infection. There is increased risk of:

- Stillbirth
- Preterm delivery
- First trimester abortion

Diagnosis

- Nasopharyngeal swabs including viral antigen rapid detection assays
- RT-PCR is the most sensitive and specific test.
- Rapid influenza diagnostic tests (RIDTs) are also available.

Management

Two classes of antivirals can be given:

1. *Neuraminidase inhibitors:* Early influenza A and B. *Oseltamivir, zanamivir,* and *peramivir*

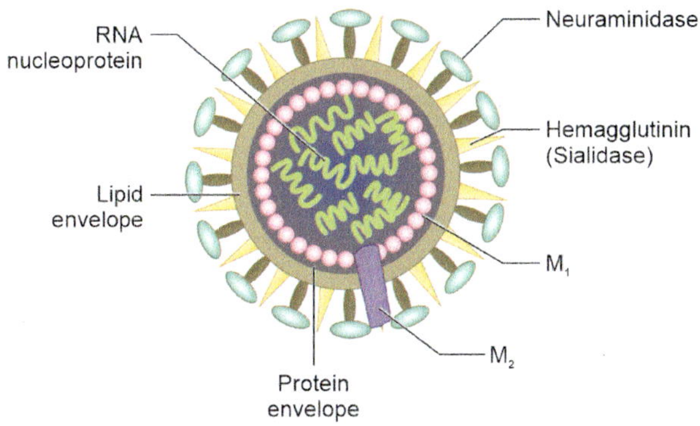

Fig. 10: Influenza virus structure.
Source: Karki G. (2020). Influenza virus-Structure, Types, Nomenclature, Transmission, Pathogenesis, Diseases, Diagnosis and Treatment. [online] Available from https://www.onlinebiologynotes.com/influenza-virus-structure-types-nomenclature-transmission-pathogenesis-diseases-diagnosis-and-treatment/. [Last accessed November, 2024]

2. *Adamantanes:* For treatment and chemoprophylaxis of influenza virus A. *Amantadine and rimantadine*

All these drugs come under category C and their safety in pregnancy is not established and thus the risk should be weighed before administration of these drugs.

COVID-19 INFECTION

The World Health Organization classified COVID-19 a global public health emergency on January 30, 2020. On the same day, the first case of COVID-19 was detected and reported in India. On March 11, 2020, the World Health Organization (WHO) labeled it a pandemic.

Coronaviruses (CoV) are a group of viruses that can cause anything from a common cold to life-threatening infections. The World Health Organization was notified on December 31st of cases of pneumonia with an unknown cause in Wuhan, China. Chinese authorities identified a novel coronavirus as the cause on January 7, 2020, and it was given the name temporary designation "2019-nCoV." The novel virus was given the name "COVID-19 virus" after that.

Severe acute respiratory syndrome coronavirus 2 (SARS-CoV-2), like other RNA viruses **(Fig. 11)**, is vulnerable to genetic evolution with the production of mutations over time, resulting in mutant variations with distinct characteristics than their parent strains. SARS-CoV-2 has several variations, including alpha, beta, gamma, delta, and omicron.

Epidemiology

The average incubation period (the time between exposure and the emergence of clinical symptoms) is 5–7 days. **Figure 12** shows the immunological effects of COVID-19 on the human body.

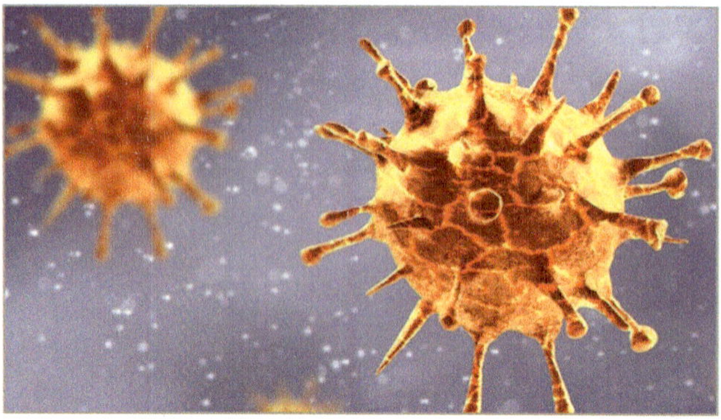

Fig. 11: Electron microscopic structure of COVID-19 virus.
Source: BBC. (2021). Covid-19: New variant 'raises R number by up to 0.7'. [online] Available from https://www.google.com/url?sa=i&url=https%3A%2F%2Fwww.bbc.com%2Fnews%2Fhealth-55507012&psig=AOvVaw3tReu319_od-05yt4429_d&ust=1644412448707000&source=images&cd=vfe&ved=0CAsQjRxqFwoTCNiOjJ6Y8PUCFQAAAAAdAAAAABAE. [Last accessed November, 2024]

By 11 days after exposure, the majority of infected people would have developed characteristics.

Pregnant women are no more likely than the general population to become infected. The virus is mainly spread by droplets and proposed by some authorities that it might be air borne. Thus, maintenance of social hygiene has been the most important step in prevention of COVID-19 infection.

Frequent washing of hands, use of face masks, gloves, social distancing, and maintaining a distance of 6 feet from others have been promoted by government as a measure to decrease the incidence of disease.

Clinical Features

The majority of persons (both pregnant and nonpregnant) may be asymptomatic or have COVID-19 infection-related respiratory symptoms. Cough, sore throat, and fever will affect the majority of pregnant women in mild-to-severe degrees. Few people may experience breathing difficulties or shortness of breath.

The WHO has classified these as symptoms of severe acute respiratory infection (SARI). If the pregnant woman has comorbid disorders such diabetes, hypertension, obesity, or respiratory disease, or if she is above the age of 50, she is more likely to develop a severe type of respiratory disease, as seen in the general population. Pregnant women with medical risk factors are more likely to develop pneumonia and severe hypoxia, or to progress to this state fast. Fatigue, malaise, body aches, and/or gastrointestinal disorders like nausea and diarrhea are common among immunocompromised and elderly pregnant women.

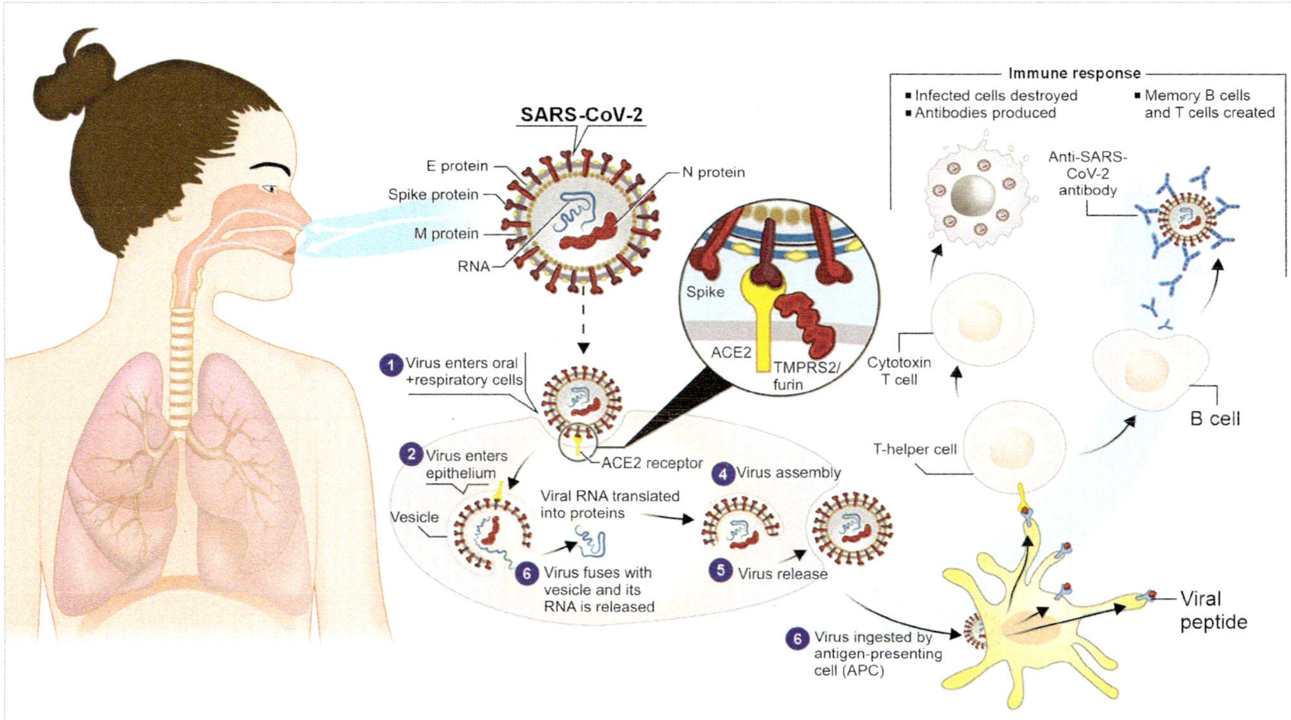

Fig. 12: COVID-19 virus and its immunological effects in human body. (ACE2: angiotensin-converting enzyme 2)

There has been increasing evidence regarding association of preeclampsia with COVID-19 viral infection. Endothelial damage is a common denominator in the pathophysiology of preeclampsia and COVID-19. Disrupted placentation is a defining feature of preeclampsia, and it leads to endothelial dysfunction and end-organ damage. Endothelial cells are infected by SARS-CoV-2, and COVID-19 lungs show endothelial cell damage, microthrombi, and angiogenesis.

Endothelial damage in both preeclampsia and COVID-19 is hypothesized to cause multiorgan dysfunction. Noncardiogenic pulmonary edema and venous thromboembolism are also more common in both conditions.

Thus, regular BP monitoring is a must in all pregnant females with current or past history of COVID-19 infection.

Diagnosis

Diagnosis is usually done by testing the nasopharyngeal sample collected using either a nasal or throat swab which is then carried to the testing facility in a liquid viral transport media.

Detection of viral antigen by rapid antigen kits takes only few minutes to hours.

Detection of viral genetic material by reverse transcription-polymerase chain reaction (RT-PCR) takes 24–48 hours depending on the testing facility. RT-PCR is the gold standard of diagnosis of COVID.

Cartridge-based nucleic acid amplification test (CB-NAAT) is also used for diagnosis in some centers.

Serological testing of IgM and IgG antibodies by enzyme-linked immunosorbent assay (ELISA) is used.

Management

- *Investigations*: Routinely, no investigation is required for mild COVID-19 cases.
- In case of persistent or worsening symptoms, following investigations can be done:
    - Complete blood count (CBC), absolute lymphocyte count, kidney function test (KFT), and liver function test (LFT)—24–48 hours
    - C-reactive protein (CRP), erythrocyte sedimentation rate (ESR), procalcitonin, interleukin 6 (IL-6), lactate dehydrogenase (LDH), ferritin, and D-dimer every 48–72 hours
    - Chest X-ray (CXR) with abdominal shield

Asymptomatic patients:

Treatment for patient with mild asymptomatic disease in home isolation **(Flowchart 2)**

Flowchart 2: Treatment algorithm of COVID-19 positive pregnant women.

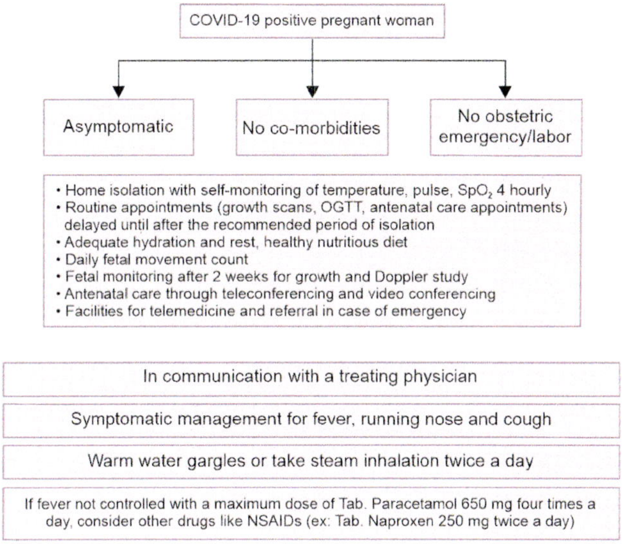

Need for admission:

- Inability to tolerate oral hydration or needed medications
- Persistent pleuritic chest pain
- Worsening shortness of breath
- Tachypnea
- New-onset confusion or lethargy
- Obstetrical symptoms, such as preterm contractions, vaginal bleeding, or decreased fetal movement
- Cyanotic lips, fingertips, or face
- Unremitting fever (>39°C) even after administering antipyretics
- Oxygen saturation <95% at rest or on exertion

Multidisciplinary approach to management of COVID including intensivist, obstetrician, and physician is mainstay. There may be need of ventilatory support and antiviral drug treatment in severe cases.

Detailed maternal and fetal monitoring is recommended.

During Labor

Fetal considerations:

- *High rate of fetal compromise:*
  - *Recommendation:* Continuous electronic fetal monitoring using cardiotocograph (CTG) in labor
- *Antenatal corticosteroids:* Between 24 and 34 weeks of gestation can be given.
- The presence of COVID-19 should not impact the mode of birth unless the woman's respiratory status necessitates an immediate delivery.

- COVID-19 is not an indication for caesarean section.
- Decision based on obstetric (fetal or maternal) indications and not COVID-19 status alone.
- Principles of labor and delivery management remain same with creation of isolation wards for suspected or confirmed cases at all levels of health care.
- Person-to-person contact should be limited.
- Time in the labor should be limited.
- For cervical ripening, mechanical ripening with a balloon catheter/ prostaglandin can be used.

For surgical procedure:
- Designated COVID OT/suspect OT
- Minimize the number of persons in the OT room
- Health care team to be in personal protective equipment (PPE)
- Minimize the movement of the team in and out of the OT during the procedure

Postpartum

Mild symptoms: Monitor vitals every 4 hours for 24 hours in cases of vaginal delivery and 48 hours in cases of caesarean delivery.

Breastfeeding:
- In hospitals, nurses trained in essential newborn care and lactation management should be provided for support.
- Mother, caretakers, and nurses should follow respiratory hygiene (triple layered surgical mask, cough, and sneeze etiquettes).
- If rooming-in is not possible, the neonate should be fed expressed breastmilk (EBM) of the mother by a nurse or trained healthy family member.
- Observe respiratory etiquettes. A healthy, asymptomatic and willing family member, negative for SARS-CoV-2, and not in direct contact with persons with suspected or confirmed infection to stay with the mother and baby to assist and provide support for breastfeeding.

Vaccination: Both Covishield and Covaxin which are available in India are recommended by FOGSI for immunization in both pregnant and breastfeeding females.

DENGUE FEVER

Dengue fever is a mosquito-borne viral disease spread by female mosquitos of the Aedes aegypti and, to a lesser extent, *Aedes albopictus* species. Chikungunya, yellow fever, and Zika viruses are all spread by mosquitos. Dengue fever is common throughout the tropics, with local differences in risk determined by climate, socioeconomic, and environmental factors.

Dengue is a disease that affects a wide range of people. This can range from asymptomatic infection (when people are unaware, they are infected) to severe flu-like symptoms in those who are afflicted. Although rare, some persons get severe dengue, which can result in a variety of consequences including severe bleeding, organ damage, and plasma leakage. When severe dengue is not treated properly, there is an increased chance of mortality.

When severe dengue is not treated properly, there is an increased chance of mortality. During dengue epidemics in the Philippines and Thailand in the 1950s, severe dengue was first identified. Severe dengue fever now affects most Latin American and Asian countries, where it is a major cause of hospitalization and death among children and adults.

Dengue fever is caused by a virus from the Flaviviridae family. There are four different serotypes of the virus that cause dengue fever (DENV-1, DENV-2, DENV-3, and DENV-4). It is thought that after recovering from an infection, person becomes immune to a disease but in dengue, the risk of severe disease increases with second infection with a different serotype.

Epidemiology

Infected female mosquitoes, typically the Aedes aegypti mosquito **(Fig. 13)**, transmit the virus to people through bites. Other Aedes species can also operate as vectors, although their role is secondary to that of Aedes aegypti.

After feeding on a DENV-infected person, the virus replicates in the mosquito midgut before migrating to secondary tissues like the salivary

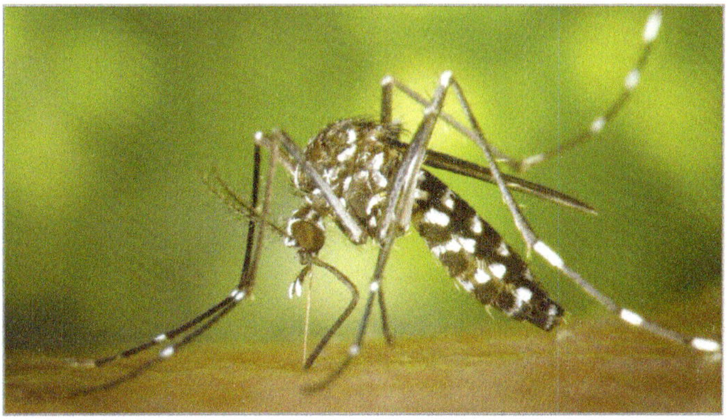

Fig. 13: Aedes mosquito.

Source: India Today. (2020). How to identify a dengue mosquito. [online] Available from https://www.google.com/url?sa=i&url=https%3A%2F%2Fwww.indiatoday.in%2Finformation%2Fstory%2Fhow-to-identify-a-dengue-mosquito-1718502-2020-09-04&psig=AOvVaw1RS5e_XliMoAsFPBWjuvaA&ust=1644403781796000&source=images&cd=vfe&ved=0CAsQjRxqFwoTCLDT5PD37_UCFQAAAAAdAAAAABAD. [Last accessed November, 2024]

glands. The mosquito can transmit the virus for the remainder of its life after it has become infected. Mosquitoes can be infected by persons who are DENV-positive.

The mosquito Aedes aegypti is thought to be the principal DENV vector. It could breed in natural containers like tree holes and bromeliads, but it has now adapted to urban habitats and now breeds primarily in man-made containers like buckets, mud pots, discarded containers and used tyres, storm water drains, and so on, making dengue an insidious disease in densely populated urban areas. Aedes aegypti feeds during the day, with peak biting periods early in the morning and just before dusk.

Clinical Features

Incubation period is 4–10 days and symptoms last for 2–7 days.

DENV may lead to a wide variety of clinical manifestations, ranging from dengue fever to dengue hemorrhagic fever (DHF), which can become more severe to cause dengue shock syndrome (DSS). DF is characterized by nonspecific symptoms such as headache, fever, myalgia, arthralgia, retrobulbar pain, nausea, vomiting, and rashes. Rash is maculopapular and blanches on pressure **(Fig. 14)**.

In addition to these signs and symptoms, DHF is marked by bleeding, thrombocytopenia, and plasma leakage, all of which are caused by increased vascular permeability. This situation can quickly develop to hypovolemic shock and, in some cases, death.

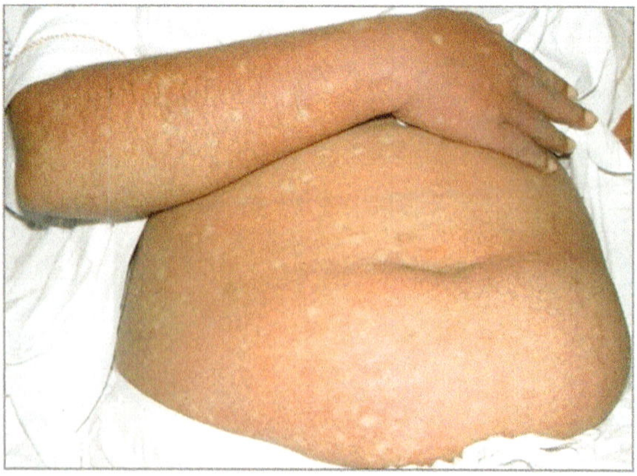

Fig. 14: Typical dengue rash.
Source: Lecturio. (2023). Dengue Virus. [online] Available from https://www.google.com/url?sa=i&url=https%3A%2F%2Fwww.lecturio.com%2Fconcepts%2Fdengue-virus%2F&psig=AOvVaw1DnKd4wUKEJ81CqnFEbTkR&ust=1644502342926000&source=images&cd=vfe&ved=0CAsQjRxqFwoTCOCfzerm8vUCFQAAAAAdAAAAABAJ. [Last accessed November, 2024]

Dengue in Pregnancy

Mosquito vectors are the principal method of transmission of DENV between people. However, there is evidence that maternal transmission is possible (from a pregnant mother to her baby). While the rate of vertical transmission appears to be modest, the risk of vertical transmission appears to be connected to when dengue occurs during pregnancy.

Antenatal complications may include premature labor, intrauterine growth retardation, fetal distress, prematurity, and risk of IUFD. Thrombocytopenia resulting from dengue may lead to antepartum hemorrhage, postpartum hemorrhage, and increased morbidity and mortality in mother.

Diagnosis

Diagnostic tests are most sensitive in 1st week of illness.

- *RT-PCR*: The gold-standard of diagnosis is isolation of virus.
- *Rapid diagnostic kit*: It tests a virus produced protein—NS1. It takes 20 minutes for diagnosis.
- *ELISA*: It is used to detect antibodies in blood of patient. IgM develops within 1 week of infection up to 3 months and signifies recent infection. IgG signifies past infection and may be present for years.

Treatment

There is no specific treatment for dengue infection.

Conservative management of dengue includes adequate hydration and inpatient management of complications. Pain management should be done by use of paracetamol (acetaminophen) and use of NSAIDs like aspirin and ibuprofen should be avoided as the antiplatelet action of these drugs might aggravate the thrombocytopenia of dengue.

The first vaccine for dengue, Dengvaxia® (CYD-TDV) developed by Sanofi Pasteur, was licensed in December 2015 and has been approved for its use by regulatory authorities in around 20 countries in November 2017. The CYD-TDV vaccination is intended for those aged 9–45 who live in endemic areas and have had at least one episode of dengue virus infection.

HERPES SIMPLEX VIRUS

The most prevalent sexually transmitted disease is genital herpes, which is caused by herpes simplex virus 2.

Herpes simplex virus 1 (HSV-1) and HSV-2 are members of a vast DNA virus family **(Fig. 15)** in which 8 are known to be infectious in humans. HSV-1 and HSV-2 are transferred by epithelial mucosal cells and skin discontinuities, and then travel to nerve tissues, where they remain latent. HSV-1 is most usually found in the trigeminal ganglia and predominates in orofacial lesions, whereas HSV-2 is most commonly found in the lumbosacral ganglia.

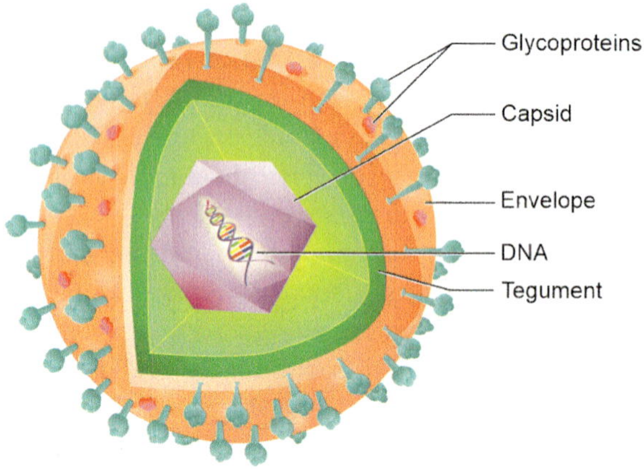

Fig. 15: Structure of herpes virus.
Source: iStock. Herpes simplex virus. [online] Available from https://www.google.com/url?sa=i&url=https%3A%2F%2Fwww.istockphoto.com%2Fillustrations%2Fherpes-simplex-virus&psig=AOvVaw3exWzLSL-vM7k_eApRGq9E&ust=1644502549961000&source=images&cd=vfe&ved=0CAsQjRxqFwoTCJihzM7n8vUCFQAAAAAdAA AAABAD. [Last accessed November, 2024]

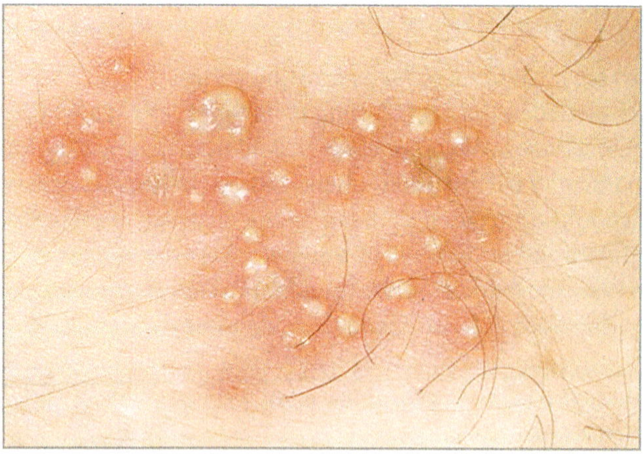

Fig. 16: Maculopapular lesions in HSV infection. (HSV: herpes simplex virus)
Source: MediFee Healthcare. Best Home Cures for Herpes. [online] Available from https://www.google.com/url?sa=i&url=https%3A%2F%2Fwww.medifee.com%2Fblog%2Fbest-home-cures-for-herpes%2F&psig=AOvVaw0f8EPmHGPHCkcMburhyrh2&ust=1644502816317000&source=images&cd=vfe&ved=0CAsQjRxqFwoTCNjXqMro8vUCFQAAAAAdAAAAABAD. [Last accessed November, 2024]

HSV-1 and HSV-2 are both capable of causing genital sores and shedding. **Figure 16** shows the typical rash that develops in herpes infection.

Epidemiology

Ethnicity, poverty, cocaine consumption, earlier initiation of sexual activity, number of lifetime sexual partners, sexual conduct, and the presence of bacterial vaginosis are all factors that influence a woman's risk of infection before pregnancy.

Herpes simplex virus has a seroprevalence of 72% in pregnant women. This refers to any infection with HSV-1 or HSV-2 that resulted in the production of antibodies.

Herpes Simplex Virus and Pregnancy

Spontaneous abortion, intrauterine growth restriction, preterm labor, and congenital and neonatal herpes infections have all been linked to HSV infection during pregnancy. Clinical therapy, on the other hand, focuses on reducing vertical transmission to the fetus, lowering the chance of newborn herpes infection.

Prior seroconversion (the presence of antibodies to both HSV-1 and -2 viruses before the pregnancy) had the lowest risk of perinatal transmission. In contrast, late-pregnancy primary or first-genital HSV infection increases the chance of neonatal infection by 30–50%, while early pregnancy infection has a risk of <1%.

Antibodies are not generated in time to reduce viral replication and shedding before labor if primary HSV infection occurs late in pregnancy.

Herpes simplex virus transmission from mother to fetus via the placenta or ascending duct is uncommon during pregnancy; 80–90% of perinatal transmission occurs during labor and delivery.

However, in the case of recurrent herpes, newborn infection with HSV can develop. At the commencement of labor, symptom recurrence that results in viral shedding is linked to a 3% chance of newborn herpes; both young age and recent infection are linked to higher viral shedding.

Neonatal Herpes

Localized skin, eye, and mouth (SEM) infection, central nervous system (CNS) with or without SEM infection, and disseminated disease are the three types of neonatal herpes infection (which carries a mortality rate in excess of 80%, if untreated). Significant neurologic impairments, blindness, convulsions, and learning problems can occur in infected babies.

Management

Asymptomatic viral shedding, clinical HSV recurrence, and caesarean delivery for recurring lesions are all reduced with suppressive antiviral medication during the last month of pregnancy. Even if suppressive medication has been utilized, a caesarean section is suggested when lesions or prodromal symptoms are evident at the commencement of labor to reduce the risk of virus exposure to the newborn.

Invasive interventions like as amniotomy, the use of fetal scalp electrodes, and surgical vaginal delivery should be avoided in women who have asymptomatic HSV in labor. This reduces the risk of the virus being transmitted to the fetus through vaginal secretions. When membranes rupture prior to the commencement of labor, active management should be explored.

The dangers of prematurity must be evaluated against the risks of HSV transmission when preterm premature rupture of the membranes (PPROM) occurs. The gestational age and clinical picture will determine the outcome in each case. For women with PPROM and a history of HSV, there is no consensus on the ideal time to deliver.

VARICELLA ZOSTER VIRUS

Varicella, usually known as chickenpox, is the varicella zoster virus's acute main illness. It is a highly contagious, self-limiting sickness that primarily affects children. It creates a widespread maculopapular to vesicular rash that starts on the face and trunk and then spreads to the limbs. It is spread via respiratory droplets or close contact. The virus takes 15 days to incubate and is spreadable 2 days before the rash appears and until all lesions have crusted or disappeared. The virus may remain latent in the dorsal root ganglia for years after an initial infection of varicella zoster, which causes chickenpox. Herpes zoster, which is more frequent in adults, is the result of reactivation.

Epidemiology

Varicella is found in 0.7 out of 1,000 pregnant women. Because varicella is primarily a childhood disease, most women are immune to it before becoming pregnant.

Primary varicella infection in pregnancy, on the other hand, is linked to severe maternal and fetal morbidity and mortality.

While the childhood sickness is self-limiting and minor, varicella pneumonia can be more severe if it occurs during pregnancy.

Varicella infection causes pneumonia in 10–20% of pregnant women, which has a death risk of up to 40%.

Clinical Features

- Fever
- Rhinitis, cough, and sore throat
- Characteristic maculopapular rash with crusting of lesions **(Fig. 17)**
- Reactivation of old lesions may present as painful blister among a single dermatomal distribution

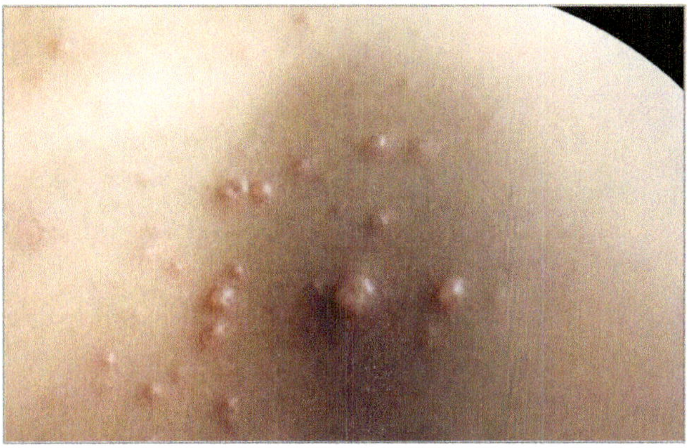

Fig. 17: Maculopapular rash of varicella infection.
Source: Bechtel KA. (2024). Pediatric Chickenpox. [online] Available from https://www.google.com/url?sa=i&url=https%3A%2F%2Femedicine.medscape.com%2Farticle%2F969773-overview&psig=AOvVaw3CsZjLyRiFj3ttetRiYFrE&ust=1644503349001000&source=images&cd=vfe&ved=0CAsQjRxqFwoTCLCLj83q8vUCFQAAAAAdAAAAABAK. [Last accessed November, 2024]

Congenital Varicella Syndrome

The development of congenital varicella syndrome is linked to fetal morbidity and mortality. Limb hypoplasia, microcephaly, hydrocephaly, cataracts, intrauterine growth restriction, and mental impairment are all symptoms of this syndrome **(Fig. 18)**.

With maternal varicella infection during the first 20 weeks of pregnancy, the risk of congenital varicella syndrome ranges from 0.4 to 2%. The reactivation of the varicella virus in utero, rather than a primary infection of the fetus, is likely to be the cause of this disease.

Neonatal infection can affect 10–20% of newborns whose moms were acutely infected between 5 days before delivery and 2 days after delivery. It occurs when the virus spreads hematogenously across the placenta in the absence of maternal antibodies. 5–10 days after delivery, infants begin to show symptoms. The clinical picture might range from cutaneous lesions to systemic sickness with a 30% death rate.

Treatment

Because no treatment regimen has been found to reduce the frequency of vertical transmission, treatment for pregnant women focuses on reducing maternal morbidity.

Tablet acyclovir is generally used in active cases with antipyretics for symptomatic management. Prevention of secondary bacterial infection is also important.

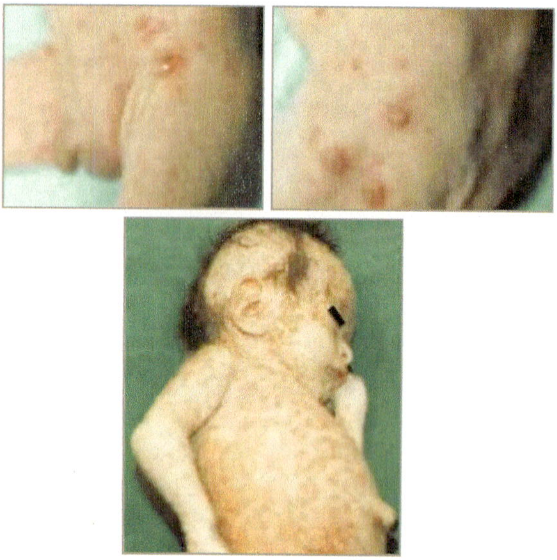

Fig. 18: Congenital varicella syndrome affected baby.
Source: https://www.google.com/url?sa=i&url=https%3A%2F%2Fwww.rrnursingschool.biz%2Fnewborns-4%2Finfo-jal.html&psig=AOvVaw3yvzIIBXB6lAyqMre2vEjj&ust=1644503433471000&source=images&cd=vfe&ved=0CAsQjRxqFwoTCIDq6Ozq8v UCFQAAAAAdAAAAABAJ.

PARASITIC DISEASES

MALARIA IN PREGNANCY

Malaria is one of the world's most common parasite infections. It is found in the majority of Asia's, South America's, and Africa's tropical countries. It could induce severe hemolytic anemia and periodic fever episodes in pregnant women. Because of the disease's high endemicity in India, it is crucial to rule out malaria in pregnant women who have a fever and anemia. Because prophylaxis and therapy for this condition are widely available, it is critical to understand the symptoms, diagnosis, consequences, and management.

Pathophysiology

Malaria is caused by infection with an obligate intracellular protozoan of the genus *Plasmodium*. Four main species are known to infect human beings:

These are:

1. *P. falciparum*
2. *P. vivax*
3. *P. malariae*
4. *P. ovale*

After the bite of a female anopheline mosquito, the erythrocyte is infected with the sporozoites of the protozoan. In a few minutes, the sporozoites invade the hepatocytes and undergo asexual multiplication to for merozoites. This is the exoerythrocytic phase. During this phase, there may be no symptoms. Once the hepatocyte undergoes rupture, the merozoites are released into the bloodstream and again invade the erythrocytes. In 48–72 hours after invasion of the erythrocyte, trophozoites and subsequently schizonts with daughter merozoites are formed. The erythrocyte will rupture and the released daughter merozoites infect other erythrocytes. Thus, the erythrocytic phase continues. Few of the merozoites undergo sexual maturation to form gametocytes. These gametocytes are infective to anopheline mosquitos. Upon ingestion of the gametocyte, it undergoes maturation in the stomach of the mosquito and further migrates to the salivary gland of the mosquito. This is how the transmission occurs through the mosquitos. **Figure 19** shows the life cycle of malaria parasite.

Other modes of transmission are:

- Through blood transfusion
- Congenital malaria
- In these modes of transmission, there is no exoerythrocytic phase. Therefore, relapses are uncommon and also long-term treatment to eradicate hepatic form is unnecessary.

Maternal Infection

The host immunity and the infecting parasite play a role in deciding the severity of infection. Of particular concern in India is the fact that pregnancy is associated with significant fall in the immunity levels due to which there is greater degree of parasitemia and clinical symptoms.

The symptoms are variable, most commonly:

- Chills
- Fever
- Headache
- Myalgia

Paroxysms of fever are characterized by rigor episodes followed by a febrile period of approximately 6 hours **(Table 1)**.

One of the main features of malaria in pregnancy is the exaggeration of anemia of pregnancy. A strong clinical suspicion is necessary if there is a combination of fever, hypersplenism, and evidence of hemolytic anemia. Folic acid deficiency can be precipitated due to high turnover of red blood cells. Lymphadenopathy is characteristically absent.

Placental insufficiency can cause second trimester abortions, fetal growth restriction, intrauterine demise, fresh stillbirth due to intrapartum asphyxia, and premature labor **(Table 2)**.

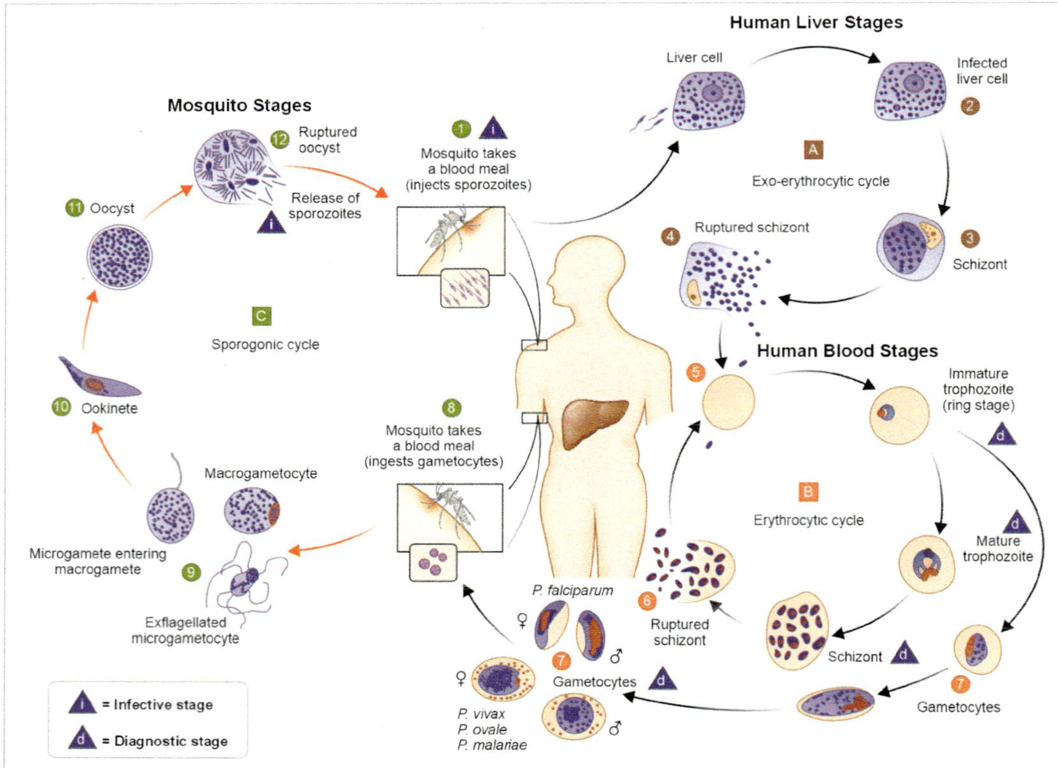

Fig. 19: Life cycle of the malaria parasite.

Source: CDC. Global Health, Division of Parasitic Diseases and Malaria. [online] Available from https://www.cdc.gov/ncezid/divisions-offices/about-dpdm.html#:~:text=The%20Division%20of%20Parasitic%20Diseases,States%20and%20around%20the%20world. [Last accessed November, 2024]

TABLE 1: Fever periodicity in malaria.

Organism	*Fever periodicity*
P. falciparum	Every 24–48 hours
P. vivax and *P. ovale*	Every 48 hours (alternate day)
P. malariae	Every 72 hours

TABLE 2: Features of malaria in pregnancy.

Nonobstetric	*Obstetric*
Fever with rigors	Midtrimester abortions
Hypersplenism	Premature labor
Hemolytic anemia	Fetal growth restriction
Folate deficiency	Intrapartum asphyxia
Convulsions (may be a feature of cerebral malaria)	Intrauterine fetal demise
Acute renal insufficiency	
Disseminated intravascular coagulation	

Congenital Malaria

The transmission of the parasite through the placenta depends on maternal immune status. There is a 30% incidence of placental malaria among women in endemic areas, however, only 10% of them are symptomatic for malaria. Demonstration of parasite in the placenta is considered more accurate than maternal blood sampling for detecting fetal affection. Direct transmission of the parasite or transmission of immunoglobulin G (IgG) from the maternal circulation is the postulated mechanisms for transmission of malaria in utero. Clinical features in the fetus may appear 2–4 weeks after birth and include fever, lethargy, anorexia, and in some cases convulsions. Hepatosplenomegaly may be absent in the initial stages but develop rather quickly once the clinical features appear.

Diagnosis

It is based on clinical suspicion and demonstration of the parasite on thick and thin blood smears. If the smears are taken during the febrile paroxysms, the chances of obtaining the parasite are higher as this is the time when the schizonts burst and merozoites are released into the circulation. Giemsa stain is used to identify the species of the parasite which will then direct the treatment required. Nowadays, rapid diagnostic kits are available for the diagnosis of malaria.

Management in Pregnancy

For prevention, a three-pronged strategy is recommended by WHO in endemic areas like Africa. This includes:

- Case management (using highly effective drugs and initiating the treatment promptly)

- Prevention with insecticide treated bed nets
- *IPTP (intermittent preventive treatment in pregnancy):* Administration of full course antimalarial treatment at regular antenatal visits. Sulfadoxine-pyrimethamine (SP) is generally used.

However, there is lack of evidence regarding the benefit of IPTP in India. Also, there is low efficacy of SP against *P. vivax*, and low levels of uptake.

Thus, the treatment protocols differ based on the severity of infection and the species of implicated parasite.

Uncomplicated Falciparum Malaria

All children and adults (except pregnant women in first trimester) should be treated with Artemisinin-based Combination Therapy (ACT). ACT should provide at least 3 days of coverage with the artemisinin derivative.

The combinations available are:

- *Artemether + Lumefantrine*
- *Artesunate + Amodiaquine*
- *Artesunate + Mefloquine*
- *Dihydroartemisinin + Piperaquine*
- *Artesunate + Sulfadoxine-Pyrimethamine*

These are available as fixed dose combinations for various weight ranges **(Table 3 to 6)**.

TABLE 3: Artemether + lumefantrine (twice daily for 3 days).

Body weight (kg)	*Dose (mg) (Am + Lf)*
5 to <15	20 + 120
15 to <25	40 + 240
25 to <35	60 + 360
≥35	80 + 480

Comments:

- Lumefantrine exposure is known to be decreased in pregnant women. Thus, treatment response should be closely monitored in them.
- This ACT is preferred because Lumefantrine is not available as a monotherapy, hence incidence of resistance is less.
- Lumefantrine is better absorbed along with fat. Hence, patients are to be instructed to take the tablets along with milk after a full meal.

TABLE 4: Artesunate + amodiaquine (daily for 3 days).

Body weight (kg)	*Dose (mg) (As + Aq)*
4.5 to <9	25 + 67.5
9 to <18	50 + 135
18 to <36	100 + 270
≥36	200 + 540

Comments:

- There is no significant change in pharmacokinetics of amodiaquine in pregnancy. Hence, dose adjustment is not required.

TABLE 5: Artesunate + mefloquine (daily for 3 days).

Body weight (kg)	*Dose (mg) (As + Aq)*
5 to <9	25 + 55
9 to <18	50 + 110
18 to <30	100 + 220
≥30	200 + 440

TABLE 6: Artesunate + sulfadoxine/pyrimethamine.

Body weight (kg)	*Artesunate dose (mg) (daily for 3 days)*	*Sulfadoxine + pyrimethamine dose (mg) (Single dose on day 1)*
5 to <10	25	250 + 12.5
10 to <25	50	500 + 25
25 to <50	100	1,000 + 50
≥50	200	1,500 + 75

Comments:

- This ACT is not available as a fixed dose combination.
- Thus, there is risk of loose distribution of artesunate tablets and treatment failures. Artesunate monotherapy is banned by WHO.
- In areas with high endemicity, there is likely high prevalence of sulfadoxine-pyrimethamine resistance.

Uncomplicated falciparum malaria in first trimester of pregnancy: The commonly used regimen for uncomplicated *P. falciparum* malaria in first trimester of pregnancy is 7 days of quinine + clindamycin (10 mg/kg body weight).

Dosages in lactation: Pharmacokinetics of most of the antimalarial drugs are not significantly altered in lactation. Tetracycline is contraindicated during lactation due to the potential adverse effects on the infant's bones and teeth. Primaquine should not be given during breastfeeding unless the breastfed infant has been checked for G6PD deficiency.

Uncomplicated P. vivax, P. ovale, and P. malariae infections:
The main objective of treatment is to target both the erythrocytic stage and the hepatic stage of the parasite, known as radical cure.

- If the species is not known with certainty, treat as uncomplicated falciparum malaria.
- In areas with chloroquine-sensitive malaria, treat uncomplicated *P. vivax, P. ovale,* and *P. malariae* infections with either ACT (except in

first trimester of pregnancy) or chloroquine (preferred in first trimester of pregnancy).

- *Dose of chloroquine*: 10 mg base/kg body weight on day 1 and day 2, followed by 5 mg base/kg body weight on day 3 of treatment.
- In areas with chloroquine-resistant malaria, treat uncomplicated *P. vivax*, *P. ovale*, and *P. malariae* infections in first trimester with quinine.
- *For preventing relapses:*
  - Weekly chemoprophylaxis with chloroquine can be considered till delivery or breastfeeding is completed.
  - Primaquine may be used only in women who are breastfeeding infants older than 6 months old, after documenting that the infant is not G6PD deficient.

Severe Malaria during Pregnancy

Second- and third-trimester pregnant women are more likely to have severe malaria compared to other adults. Pulmonary edema and hypoglycemia may complicate these cases. Intrauterine fetal demises and preterm labor are often seen. Maternal mortality with severe malaria is in the range of 50%.

Parenteral artesunate in full dose should be immediately started. If artesunate is not available, artemether IM can be given. If this is also not available, treatment may be started with Quinine till artesunate is made available.

Severe vivax malaria may present with anemia, thrombocytopenia, pulmonary edema, cerebral malaria, pancytopenia, jaundice, splenic rupture, acute kidney injury, and shock. All these need to be concomitantly treated along with achieving radical cure through parenteral antimalarials.

Conclusion

Malaria is a common, mostly benign, and frequently under diagnosed condition in pregnancy.

Simple combination therapies are available which help to achieve complete cure and prevent maternal and perinatal morbidity and mortality.

Adherence to treatment, monitoring of clinical response, and high suspicion of drug resistance are imperative to avoid complications, relapse, and recrudescence.

LEISHMANIASIS

Organism and its Life Cycle

Leishmania is obligate intracellular protozoan that infects people in four different species.

Throughout the body, *L. donovani* predominantly infects reticuloendothelial cells. It causes the disease kala-azar and is found

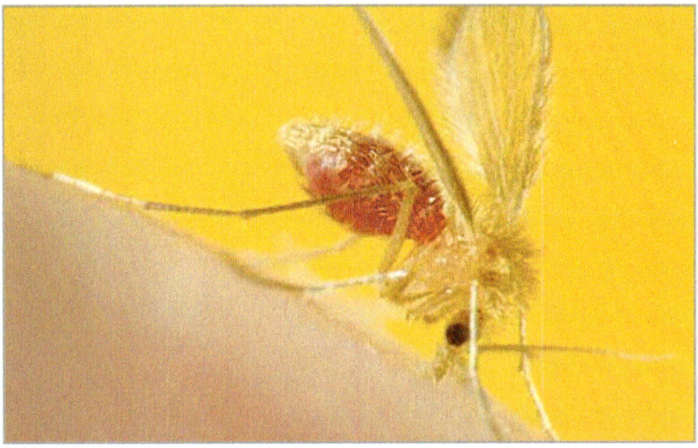

Fig. 20: Sandfly phlebotomus species.
Source: CDC. Global Health, Division of Parasitic Diseases and Malaria DPDx.

throughout Asia, Europe, Africa, India, and areas of Central and South America in the Western Hemisphere. The sandfly (Phlebotomus) is the primary vector, and a number of tiny animals serve as key reservoirs for the illness. The classic form of cutaneous leishmaniasis is Leishmania tropica (Oriental sore). *L. braziliensis* and *L. mexicana* (New World leishmaniasis) cause ulcers of the oral and nasal mucosa, usually after a primary skin ulcer has developed. These mucosal ulcers often advance to the point where the nose is completely destroyed.

The bite of sandflies belonging to the genus *Phlebotomus* **(Fig. 20)** transmits the various species of leishmania. Sandflies pick up the protozoan either directly from contaminated skin or by consuming parasites that circulate in the reservoir host's blood. Leishmania evolves into a human-infectious flagellate (promastigote) in the sandfly. The promastigote enters macrophages of the reticuloendothelial system (*L. donovani*) or histiocytes in dermal tissue (cutaneous leishmaniasis) after being inoculated into a human host, where it transforms into amastigote forms and divides by binary fission. After proliferation, offspring amastigotes infect surrounding histiocytes or spread across the reticuloendothelial system in the case of visceral leishmaniasis. **Figure 21** shows the life cycle of leishmania.

Clinical Manifestations

Visceral Leishmaniasis

The incubation period for the visceral version of the disease can range from 2 weeks to 18 months. The start of fever, which usually consists of two daily spikes, might be rapid or gradual. It lasts for 1–6 weeks before disappearing and reappearing at unpredictable intervals during the sickness.

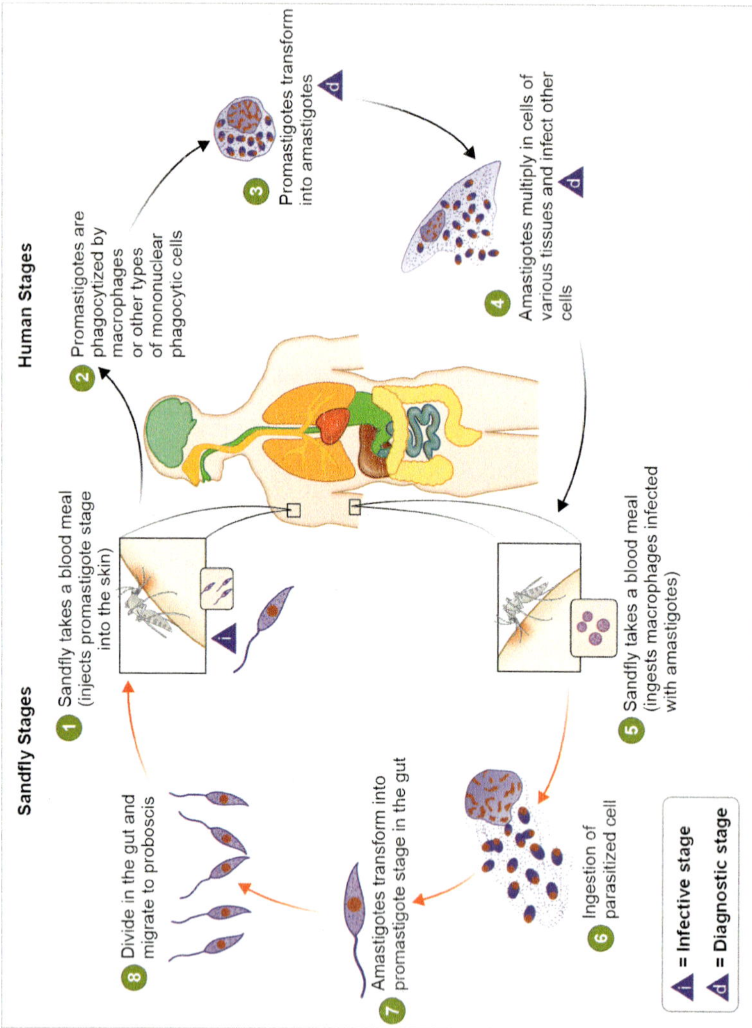

Fig. 21: Life cycle of leishmania.

Source: CDC. Global Health, Division of Parasitic Diseases and Malaria DPDx.

Splenomegaly, lymphadenopathy, and hepatomegaly are common physical findings, as are symptoms of portal hypotension and edema. Anemia and thrombocytopenia with hypergammaglobulinemia are common, and they are commonly accompanied by hemorrhage. The skin gets gray as the disease progresses, and light-skinned people may notice hyperpigmentation. The majority of individuals with visceral leishmaniasis are severely disabled and infertile, yet if pregnancy occurs during the early stages of the disease, there is a chance of intrauterine fetal infection. There has been a case of congenital leishmaniasis. Increased fetal wasting is almost invariably linked to infection with *L. donovani.*

Cutaneous Leishmaniasis

L. tropica, *L. braziliensis*, and *L. mexicana* all have comparable clinical symptoms of cutaneous leishmaniasis. At the site of inoculation, the disease begins as a pruritic crimson papule. The lesion usually expands to a diameter of 2 cm or greater and ulcerates 2–6 months after the vector bite. Over the course of a year, these lesions usually recover. In *L. mexicana* and *L. braziliensis* infection, however, severe mucocutaneous lesions can occur years after the main disease has healed.

Diagnosis

The presence of leishmanial organisms in stained preparations of blood, bone marrow, lymph nodes, or material obtained by splenic puncture is used to diagnose visceral leishmaniasis. Serologic tests are not always accurate, and in kala-azar patients, the leishmanin skin test is usually negative. Suspicion and evidence of the organism in scrapings or by culture are used to diagnose cutaneous leishmaniasis. The leishmanin skin test is normally positive during the main lesion stage, but in rare cases of disseminated cutaneous leishmaniasis, it may become negative. For the diagnosis of leishmaniasis, newer diagnostic modalities based on polymerase chain reaction (PCR) technology are being developed. **Figure 22** shows amastigote forms of leishmania.

Treatment

Because there is no known harm to the mother or fetus from cutaneous leishmaniasis, treatment should be avoided during pregnancy and postponed until after delivery. Patients with visceral leishmaniasis, on the other hand, must be treated right away, regardless of whether or not they are pregnant. The treatment of choice for all kinds of leishmaniasis is sodium antimony gluconate (Pentostam). The adult dose for visceral leishmaniasis is 20 mg/kg/day given intravenously or intramuscularly for 30 days. The dose for cutaneous leishmaniasis is 0.6 g intramuscularly given for 10 days. Amphotericin B, 0.25–1 mg/kg intravenously daily or every other day for

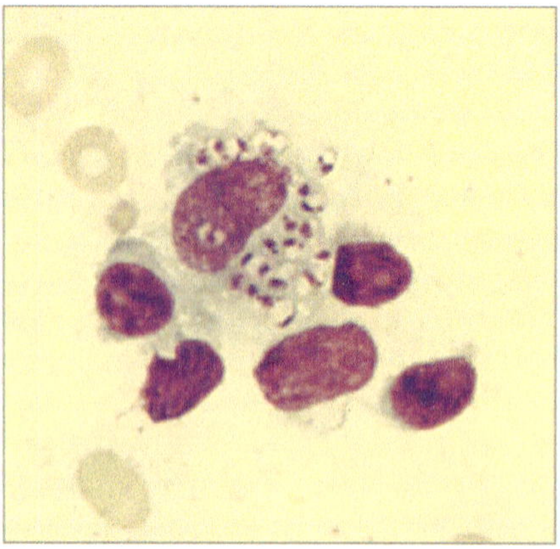

Fig. 22: Leishmania species amastigotes in a Giemsa-stained tissue scraping.
Source: CDC. Global Health, Division of Parasitic Diseases and Malaria DPDx.

up to 8 weeks, should be given to patients who do not react to antimonials. Antimonials' toxicity during pregnancy is unknown.

CONCLUSION

Viral, bacterial, parasitic infections can lead to fever in pregnancy. Prompt clinical assessment and laboratory investigations can aid us to come to a diagnosis. Infections are also associated with increased maternal and perinatal morbidity.

SUGGESTED READING

1. Armistead B, Oler E, Adams Waldorf K, Rajagopal L. The Double Life of Group B Streptococcus: Asymptomatic Colonizer and Potent Pathogen. J Mol Biol. 2019;431(16):2914-31.
2. Avantor. Salmonella typhimurium Slide. [online] Available from https://pr.vwr.com/store/product/8886425/salmonella-typhimurium-slide. [Last accessed November, 2024]
3. Banerjee D. Possible congenital infection in kala-azar. J Indian Med Assoc. 1955;24:433.
4. Basurko C, Carles G, Youssef M, Guindi WE. Maternal and foetal consequences of dengue fever during pregnancy. Eur J Obstet Gynecol Reprod Biol. 2009;147(1):29-32.
5. Bryceson ADM. Diffuse cutaneous leishmaniasis in Ethiopia. Trans R Soc Trop Med Hyg. 1970;64:369.
6. Centers for Disease Control and Prevention. Leptospirosis. [online] Available from https://www.cdc.gov/leptospirosis/index.html. [Last accessed November, 2024]
7. Chavan N, Mirza H, Sonawane P, Iqbal U. Feto-maternal outcome in COVID-19 positive patients with hypertensive disorders in pregnancy. Int J Reprod Contracept Obstet Gynecol. 2021;10(5):1846-50.
8. Deborggraeve S, Laurent T, Espinosa D, Van der Auwera G, Mbuchi M, Wasunna M, et al. A simplified and standardized polymerase chain reaction format for the diagnosis of leishmaniasis. J Infect Dis. 2008;198:1565-72.

9. Gaillard F. Pulmonary tuberculosis. Case study. [online] Available from https://radiopaedia.org/cases/8632. [Last accessed November, 2024]
10. Gandhi A, Ganatra A, Tank P. (2020). FOGSI's GCPR on Pregnancy with COVID-19 Infection. Version 2.0. [online] Available from https://www.fogsi.org/wp-content/uploads/2024/11/fogsi_gcpr_on_pregnancy_with_COVID_19_version_2.pdf. [Last accessed November, 2024]
11. Haake DA, Levett PN. Leptospirosis in humans. Curr Top Microbiol Immunol. 2015;387:65-97.
12. Jameson J. Harrison's principles of internal medicine, 20th edition. New York, NY: McGraw-Hill Education; 2018.
13. Karki G. (2020). Influenza virus-Structure, Types, Nomenclature, Transmission, Pathogenesis, Diseases, Diagnosis and Treatment. [online] Available from https://www.onlinebiologynotes.com/influenza-virus-structure-types-nomenclature-transmission-pathogenesis-diseases-diagnosis-and-treatment/. [Last accessed November, 2024]
14. Laison R, Shaw JJ. Epidemiology and ecology of leishmaniasis in Latin America. Nature. 1978;273:595.
15. Larkin GL, Thuma PE. Congenital malaria in a hyperendemic area. Am J Trop Med Hyg. 1991;45:587.
16. Low GC, Cook WE. A congenital case of kala-azar. Lancet. 1926;211:1209.
17. McConnell A. (2020). Fever, Abdominal pain, Constipation and Mary. [online] Available from https://litfl.com/fever-abdominal-pain-constipation-and-mary/. [Last accessed November, 2024]
18. Nyirjesy P, Kavasy T, Axelrod P, Fisher PR. Malaria during pregnancy: Neonatal morbidity and mortality and the efficacy of chloroquine prophylaxis. Clin Infect Dis. 1993;16:127.
19. Pouliot SH, Xiong X, Harville E, Paz-Soldan V, Tomashek KM, Breart G, et al. Maternal Dengue and Pregnancy Outcomes: A Systematic Review. Obstet Gynecol Surv. 2010;65(2):107-18.
20. Ramana KV, Reddy KM, Palange P, Rao BM, Rao SD. Cerebral Abscess Caused by Streptococcus spp in a Patient with Chronic Suppurative Otitis Media (CSOM). Am J Infect Dis Microbiol. 2014;2(5):131-7.
21. Sampaio SAP, Godoy JT, Paiva L, Dillon NL, da Lacaz CS. The treatment of American (mucocutaneous) leishmaniasis with amphotericin B. Arch Dermatol. 1960;82:627.
22. Siler JF, Hall MW, Hitchens AP. Dengue: Its history, epidemiology, mechanism of transmission, etiology, clinical manifestations, immunity and prevention. Manila: Bureau of Science; 1926.
23. The Rockefeller University. (2018). Study identifies genetic mutation responsible for tuberculosis vulnerability. [online] Available from https://www.rockefeller.edu/news/24686-study-identifies-genetic-mutation-responsible-tuberculosis-vulnerability/. [Last accessed November, 2024]
24. Waggoner JJ, Gresh L, Vargas MJ, Ballesteros G, Tellez Y, Soda KJ, et al. Viremia and Clinical Presentation in Nicaraguan Patients Infected With Zika Virus, Chikungunya Virus, and Dengue Virus. Clin Infect Dis. 2016;63(12):1584-90.
25. Williams J, Cunningham F, Leveno K, Bloom S, Hauth J, Gilstrap L, et al. Obstetrics, 25th edition. Estados Unidos: McGraw-Hill; 2005.
26. World Health Organization. Guidelines for the treatment of malaria. Geneva: WHO; 2015.

Local Causes

INTRODUCTION

Local causes of infection can be intra-amniotic infection, skin and soft tissue infection and vaginal infection.

INTRA-AMNIOTIC INFECTIONS

It is infection of liquor and intra-amniotic sac during pregnancy and is also called as chorioamnionitis.

It is commonly present with prolonged labor, preterm premature rupture of membrane (PPROM), premature rupture of membrane (PROM), or with very old macerated IUD.

Incidence is overall 4–10% of all deliveries. Clinically, patient will have fever, uterine tenderness, leukocytosis, fetal tachycardia, and maternal tachycardia.

Chorioamnionitis is histologically characterized by inflammatory cell infiltration of the membranes that are layers of amnion and chorion.

Histologic chorioamnionitis occurs more frequently than clinical sepsis and is usually not associated with clinical signs.

Etiology

Amniotic fluid is sterile in nature.

It occurs from an ascending infection of cervical or vaginal microbial flora, bacteremia, or iatrogenic causes.

Most cases result from ascending infection, rupture of membranes. With the onset of labor or rupture of membranes, bacteria indigenous to the vaginal tract ascend into the uterine cavity. It can also spread via hematogenous route.

Iatrogenic introduction of bacteria can occur during various procedures like cervical cerclage, amniocentesis, and cordocentesis, the risk of iatrogenic arterial injuries (IAI) is small.

Risk Factors

These include PROM, preterm, prolonged labor, maternal infections, and severe anemia.

Prolonged Labor

Prolonged ruptured membranes, prolonged labor, multiple vaginal examinations, and internal fetal monitoring are consistently associated with IAI.

Prelabor rupture of membranes with excess vaginal examinations increased the risk of chorioamnionitis by fivefold.

Multiple vaginal examinations, maternal colonization with group B streptococcus, prior events of abortion, and prolonged second stage of labor are risk factors for IAI.

Abnormal Vaginal Flora

An association between bacterial vaginosis (BV) and intra-amniotic infections exists.

It is based on:

- Epidemiologic studies showing an increased risk of IAI
- Presence of BV can frequently be associated with increased risk of infection
- The recovery of BV-associated microorganisms from chorioamnionitis among women with histologic chorioamnionitis and preterm delivery

Thus, BV is associated both with IAI and with preterm birth.

Diagnosis

Diagnosis of chorioamnionitis must be promptly made according to clinical correlation and higher antibiotics should be promptly started.

Early diagnosis of intra-amniotic infection is important so that timely treatment and interventions are done.

Early diagnosis is difficult because the clinical signs and symptoms of IAI occur late and are neither sensitive nor specific, a high index of suspicion is important, along with adjunctive laboratory tests.

Criteria for the clinical diagnosis of intra-amniotic infection:

- Maternal fever 37.8°C

Two or more of the following:

- Maternal leukocytosis 15,000/mm^3
- Uterine tenderness
- Maternal tachycardia >100 beats per minute
- Fetal tachycardia >160 beats per minute
- Malodorous amniotic fluid

No other apparent source of infection.

Other laboratory tests like C-reactive protein (CRP) or inflammatory markers help to make the diagnosis. These include measurement of CRP, examination of amniotic fluid leukocytes or bacteria, amniotic fluid culture, and amniotic fluid glucose concentrations, amniotic fluid leukocyte esterase, bacterial organic acids by gas-liquid chromatography, various amniotic fluid or vaginal cytokines (e.g., interleukins 2, 4, 6, granulocyte colony-stimulating factor, and tumor necrosis factor-alpha), matrix metalloproteinase-9, and lactoferrin.

Cytokine measurement is expensive and generally not clinically available.

Although all have reasonable sensitivity, specificity, and predictive value, none is sufficiently sensitive or specific to be used independently of clinical features in the diagnosis of IAI.

The range of the predictive values observed in these studies may depend, in part, on both the variable prevalence of IAI in the study population and on the cross-sectional nature of the studies, because amniotic fluid is obtained only at a single time during a temporally progressive infection. Animal models that allow longitudinal sampling of amniotic fluid after infection are helpful to delineate the natural progression of laboratory markers in infection.

Treatment

It is frequently a polymicrobial infection, with both facultative and anaerobic microorganisms, and broad-spectrum antibiotics are indicated.

Even if group B streptococci and *E. coli* account for only about 20% of isolates, these two pathogens are responsible for 60–70% of cases of neonatal sepsis and meningitis.

Antibiotic therapy should be begun in the intrapartum period, as soon as the diagnosis is confirmed, as intrapartum antibiotics improve the neonatal outcome.

A combination of IV ampicillin (2 g 6 hours) and an aminoglycoside such as gentamicin, 1.5 mg/kg intravenously every 8 hours, is most commonly used in clinical practice.

These agents also provide limited anaerobic coverage. Thus, clindamycin, 900 mg intravenously every 8 hours, is added to this regimen for patients with IAI who undergo caesarean delivery to prevent postpartum endomyometritis.

For most infections, single-agent therapy with a broad-spectrum antibiotic is equally efficacious.

Recommended intravenous regimens include injection cefotetan (2 g every 12 hours), injection piperacillin or mezlocillin (4 g every 6 hours).

Because of the greater risk of postpartum endomyometritis after caesarean delivery, the chosen antibiotic regimen should be continued until the patient has been afebrile and symptoms have resolved for at least 24 hours. **Table 7** describes antibiotic treatment for intra-amniotic infection.

Antibiotics should be started as soon as the diagnosis of chorioamnionitis is made.

Delivery is essential for treatment, and prompt action to effect delivery should be begun at the time of diagnosis, but caesarean should be reserved for usual obstetric indications.

When caesarean delivery is necessary, extraperitoneal caesarean offers no benefit to reduce the risk of postpartum sepsis.

Continuous electronic fetal monitoring is necessary during intrapartum period for delivery. The combination of villous edema, hyperthermia, and fetal infection may contribute to fetal acidosis.

TABLE 7: Antibiotic treatment of intra-amniotic infection.

Ampicillin +	2 g IV every 6 hours
Gentamicin	1.5 mg/kg IV every 8 hours,
	or 4.5 mg/kg IV every 24 hours
If delivered by caesarean, add clindamycin 900 mg IV every 8 hours	
Ampicillin/sulbactam	3.0 g IV every 6 hours
Piperacillin	4.0 g IV every 6 hours
Mezlocillin	4.0 g IV every 6 hours
Cefotetan	2.0 g IV every 12 hours

Persistent fetal tachycardia may portend a hemodynamically unstable neonate, and personnel skilled in neonatal resuscitation should be present.

Maternal complications include:
- Dysfunctional labor
- Increased operative interference
- Maternal sepsis and death
- Disseminated intravascular coagulation (DIC)

The rate of caesarean delivery is increased approximately threefold, to 35–40% mainly as a result of dystocia.

Complications associated with caesarean delivery, including blood loss, wound infection, and endomyometritis, are also increased.

Neonatal Outcome

Neonates (term) have increased risks of:
- A low Apgar score
- Pneumonia
- Sepsis

Preterm neonates have higher morbidity and mortality. Complications in preterm neonates include respiratory distress syndrome, intraventricular hemorrhage, and neurologic deficits.

It can also cause paraventricular leukomalacia in preterm or low-birth weight neonates.

SKIN AND SOFT TISSUE INFECTIONS

Skin is organ with largest surface area with multiple functions like protection of internal organs, thermoregulatory function and endocrine, apocrine function. It has rich vascular and neural supply and it is in direct contact with external environment. So, any break in skin layer will lead to increased susceptibility of infections.

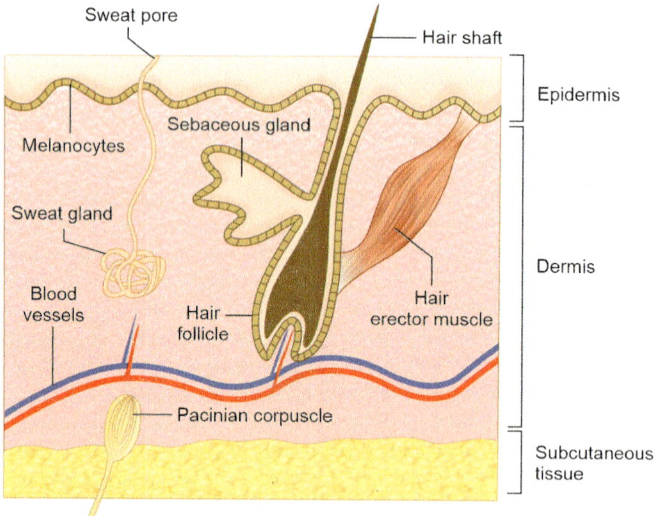

Fig. 23: Cross-section of skin.

Pregnancy itself does not increase risk of skin infections; therefore, risk of infection is same as with nonpregnant female.

Cross-section of skin **(Fig. 23):**

Types of lesions in skin infection:

- Minor skin lesions
- Cellulitis
- Folliculitis
- Boils or furuncles
- Carbuncles
- Erysipelas
- Deep tissue abscess

Sites of infection according to layers of skin **(Fig. 24)**:

Modes of infection:

- *Exogenous infection:* Due to minor trauma, breakage in layers of skin, ulcers
- *Endogenous spread:* It can be secondary to systemic infections or spread from hematogenous route.

Clinical Presentation

These are relatively rare causes of pyrexia in pregnant woman. Clinically patient will have history of skin infection (acute or chronic), history of fever, and, on investigations, total leukocytes may be raised and clinical presentation is very much similar with nonpregnant patients of similar etiology. It can be

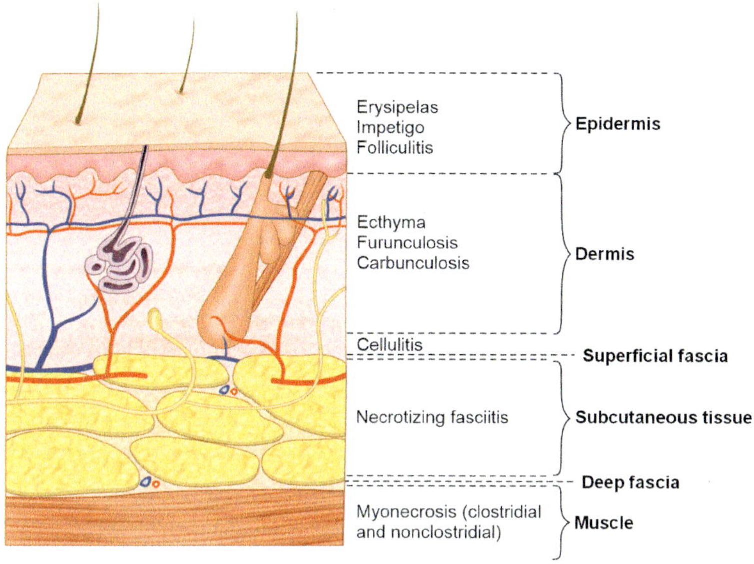

Fig. 24: Sites of infection according to layers of skin.

associated with cellulitis. Lesions can be found over extremities, breasts, buttocks, or groin.

Clinical Features

These are local pain, warmth, skin discoloration, swelling, and visible skin lesions.

Patients with systemic infection can be presented with features of shock, i.e., endotoxin shock and should be managed promptly.

Investigations

- Complete blood count
- Erythrocyte sedimentation rate (ESR) and CRP
- Gram staining of infected site
- Skin biopsy if leprosy patch
- Other investigations to rule out systemic and infectious causes of fever

Treatment

According to extent of lesion and clinical presentation, patient is considered for admission.

- Antibiotics to be started according to results of culture sensitivity.
- Penicillin group antibiotics must be started till culture sensitivity report is awaited.
- IV antibiotics should be considered for methicillin-resistant *Staphylococcus aureus* (MRSA) infection.

- Vancomycin is started for MRSA or in patients with hospital-acquired infections.
- Complicated soft tissue infections may require surgical interventions.
- Incision and drainage under local anesthesia can be safely done for abscess.
- Dermatologist should be involved while managing complicated skin lesions with chronic course or with uncertain diagnosis.

GENITAL INFECTIONS/VAGINAL INFECTIONS

Genital or vaginal infections as a causative factor of pyrexia in pregnancy are rare. It is because of formation of thick cervical mucus plug and also estrogenic as well as progestogenic effect on vaginal epithelium making it thick and stratified. Therefore, most of the times vaginitis, if present, it is pre-existing. Vaginitis or genital infections have multifactorial etiology, and pregnancy does not increase risk of vaginitis.

Defensive factors to prevent genital infections:

- *Vulval defense:* Apposition of labia majora
    - Apocrine glands and secretions from Bartholin's gland
- *Vaginal defense:* Stratified squamous epithelium of vagina
    - Vaginal rugosity
    - Doderlein's bacilli causing acidic pH
- *Cervical defense:* Mucus plug
    - Racemose glands
- *Uterine defense:* Cyclic shedding of endometrium
    - Closure of tubal ostia
- *Tubal defense:* Mucus plicae and cilia
    - Tubal peristalsis

Causative agents:

- *Gram-positive cocci: Staphylococcus*
    - Anaerobic streptococci, peptostreptococci, and clostridium group
- *Gram-negative cocci: Escherichia coli, Pseudomonas, Klebsiella, Neisseria* group
    - Bacteroides fragilis
- *Acid-fast bacilli: Mycobacterium tuberculosis*
- *Fungal agents: Candida albicans*
- *Parasitic agents:* Trichomonas vaginalis

Out of these, the most common causes of vaginitis include candidial moniliasis, trichomoniasis and bacterial vaginosis. All ANC patients should be enquired about history of sexually transmitted diseases as they can have effect on fetomaternal outcome as chances of spontaneous abortions, preterm labor, intrauterine growth restriction (IUGR), prelabor rupture of membranes, and puerperal infections are raised in such cases.

Bacterial Vaginosis

It is termed as "Vaginosis" as it is per se not an infection but altered growth of vaginal resident flora. Normally, Doderlein bacteria predominate in vaginal flora and keep intravaginal pH acidic. Overgrowth of other commensals leads to alteration of vaginal pH.

Main causative agent in such cases is Gardnerella vaginalis.

Risk factors are similar to those of other causes of vaginitis. It can cause spontaneous abortions, preterm labor, or premature rupture of membranes in pregnant woman so antenatal diagnosis and management is very important.

Clinical Features

Appearance of tissue:

- Normal,
- Homogenous PV
- Discharge that is adherent to vaginal walls
- It can be malodorous

Diagnosis

- Vaginal pH—4.5 (alkaline)
- Presence of clue cells (vaginal epithelial cells with adhered bacteria at periphery)
- Few lactobacilli may be seen.
- Whiff test—positive (fishy smell on pouring 10% KOH)

For diagnosis of bacterial vaginosis, Amsel's criteria are used, i.e., three out of four criteria must be met from following:

- Alkaline vaginal pH
- Positive whiff test
- Presence of clue cells
- Characteristic vaginal discharge

Candidiasis

It is also called vaginal moniliasis. It is most common form of vaginitis, also common immunocompromised states like uncontrolled diabetes, HIV positive patients, and patients taking antibiotics for prolonged periods. It is also common in pregnancy due to change in pH of vagina and immune status of the mother.

Causative agents include *Candida albicans, Candida glabrata,* and other forms.

Clinical Features

Patients come with history of profound vulval itching, thick curdy white discharge. Many times, associated history of diabetes or immune compromised state may be associated.

On examination:

- Vulval erythema
- Vulval swelling is present
- Thick curdy white discharge is present on per speculum examination.

Diagnosis

- Most of the times diagnosis is based on clinical findings.
- Vaginal pH is normal.
- Microscopic examination of wet mount KOH shows—presence of pseudohyphae and presence of mycelia
- Tangles or budding yeast
- Whiff test is negative
- Culture on Nickerson media and sabouraud dextrose agar shows pseudohyphae and presence of budding yeast.

Trichomoniasis

It is common form of vaginitis caused by protozoa trichomonas vaginalis **(Fig. 25)**. It affects both male and female partners and in male, it can be presented as balanitis or urethritis.

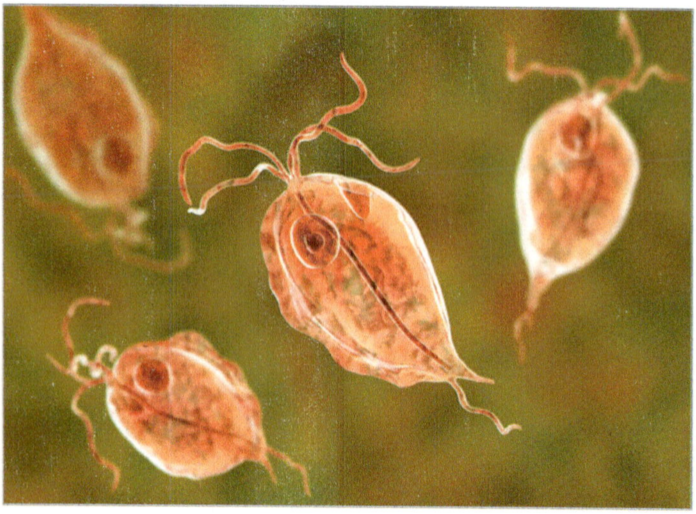

Fig. 25: *Trichomonas vaginalis.*

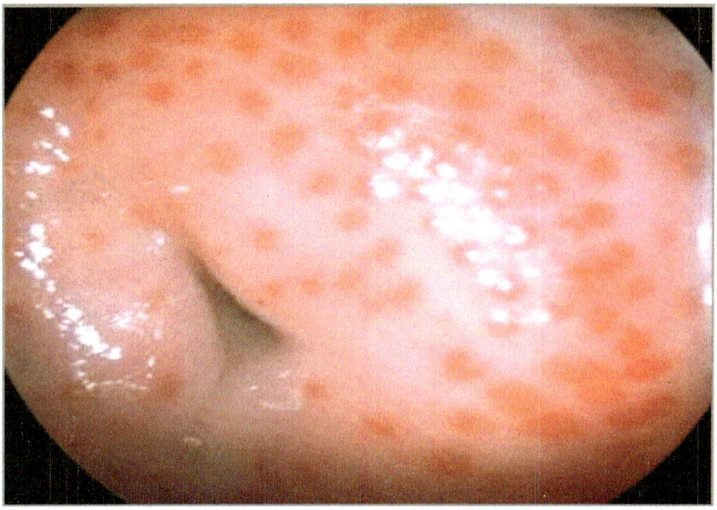

Fig. 26: Strawberry appearance of cervix.

Trichomonas vaginalis is unicellular, uniflagellate protozoa with undulating membrane.

It has axoplasm and undulating membrane with unidirectional mobility.

Clinical Features

- Both male and female partners are usually symptomatic.
- Foul-smelling vaginal discharge which is greenish white in color is seen.
- Intense vulval itching is present.
- Nocturnal itching is more common.
- On per speculum examination, strawberry cervix and strawberry vagina are pathognomonic of trichomoniasis **(Fig. 26)**.
- Hanging drop test is positive for motile organism.

Treatment of Vaginal Infections

Vaginitis prevention:

- Personal and local hygiene
- Avoid clothes that hold in heat and moisture. Nylon undergarments, tight jeans or trousers, gym shorts and leggings that do not allow passage of air, and pantyhose without a cotton panel can lead to yeast infections.
- Condoms are the best way to prevent sexually transmitted diseases.
- PAP smear screening for all antenatal patients if not done earlier
- **Table 8** highlights the treatment regimen for BV, vulvovaginal candidiasis, and trichomoniasis.

TABLE 8: Treatment regimen for bacterial vaginosis, vulvovaginal candidiasis, and trichomoniasis.

Initial regimens	*Alternative regimens*	*Pregnancy*	*Recurrence*	*Treatment of sex partners*
Bacterial vaginosis:				
Metronidazole 400 mg orally thrice daily for 7 days* or Metronidazole 0.75% gel one full applicator (5 g) intravaginally daily for 5 days or Clindamycin 2% cream, one full applicator (5 g) intravaginally at bedtime for 7 days[†]	Tinidazole 2 g orally once daily for 2 days or Tinidazole, 1 g orally once daily for 5 days or Clindamycin, 300 mg orally twice daily for 7 days or Clindamycin, 100 mg intravaginally at bedtime for 3 days	Metronidazole, 400 mg orally thrice daily for 7 days	*First recurrence:* Retrial of same regimen or Trial of alternative initial regimen *Multiple recurrences:* Metronidazole 0.75% gel, intravaginally twice weekly for 4–6 months	Routine treatment of sex partners is not recommended
Vulvovaginal candidiasis:				
Topical azole therapy[‡] or Fluconazole 150 mg orally, single dose	–	Topical azole therapy applied intravaginally for 7 days	*To achieve mycologic cure[$]:* Topical azole therapy for 7–14 days or Fluconazole 150 mg orally every third day for three doses *For maintenance:* Oral fluconazole (100 mg, 150 mg, or 200 mg) weekly for 6 months; consider topical treatment if oral is not feasible	Routine treatment of sex partners is not recommended unless the partner is symptomatic

Contd...

Contd...

Initial regimens	***Alternative regimens***	***Pregnancy***	***Recurrence***	***Treatment of sex partners***
Trichomoniasis:				
Metronidazole 2 g orally, single or divided dose on the same day or Tinidazole, 2 g orally, single dose	Metronidazole, 400 mg orally thrice daily for 7 days	Metronidazole 2 g orally, single dose in any stage of pregnancy	• Differentiate persistent or recurrent infection from reinfection[‖] • *If metronidazole, 2 g single dose fails:* Trial of metronidazole 400 mg thrice daily for 7 days • *If metronidazole 400 mg thrice daily for 7 days fails:* Trial of metronidazole 2 g daily for 7 days • *If above regimens fail:* Consider susceptibility testing	• Concurrent treatment of sex partners is recommended • Advise refraining from intercourse until partners are treated and symptom-free

Note:

* Because of disulfiram-like reaction, alcohol should be avoided for at least 24 hours after completing oral regimen.

[†] Clindamycin cream is oil-based and can weaken latex condoms and diaphragms for at least 5 days after use.

[‡] Topical azole creams and suppositories may be oil-based and can weaken latex condoms and diaphragms.

[$] *For Candida albicans* infection. Consider culture to exclude nonalbicans infection. If nonalbicans infection is present, consider first-line therapy with 7–14 days of a nonfluconazole azole agent. If infection recurs, prescribe 600 mg of boric acid in a gelatin capsule intravaginally once daily for 2 weeks. Boric acid may also be used with initial induction therapy followed by monthly maintenance therapy for recurrent albicans infection as per the Society of Obstetricians and Gynaecologists of Canada recommendations.

[‖] Follow-up with retesting as early as 2 weeks but within 3 months is recommended because rates of reinfection are high.

CONCLUSION

Local as well as systemic causes can lead to pyrexia during pregnancy. Maternal and perinatal morbidity associated with infections, can be decreased by prompt diagnosis and treatment.

SUGGESTED READING

1. Beigi RH, Austin MN, Meyn LA, Krohn MA, Hillier SL. Antimicrobial resistance associated with the treatment of bacterial vaginosis. Am J Obstet Gynecol. 2004;191(4):1124-9.
2. Chaijareenont K, Sirimai K, Kiriwat O. Accuracy of Nugent's score and each Amsel's criteria in the diagnosis of bacterial vaginosis. J Med Assoc Thai. 2004;87:1270-4.
3. Egan ME, Lipsky MS. Diagnosis of vaginitis. Am Fam Physician. 2000; 62(5):1095-104.
4. Gilbert GL. Routine antenatal screening and prenatal diagnosis of vertically transmissible infection. Baillieres Clin Obstet Gynaecol. 1993;7:1-23.
5. Goldenberg RL, Hauth JC, Andrews WW. Intrauterine infection and Preterm Delivery. NEJM. 2000;342:1500-7.
6. Hainer BL, Gibson MV. Vaginitis. Am Fam Physician. 2011;83(7):807-15.
7. Hurley R. Fever and infectious diseases. In: de Swiet (Ed). Medical disorders in obstetric practice. Oxford: Blackwell Scientific Publications; 1995.
8. Hurley R. Infection in pregnancy. In: Chamberlain G (Ed). Turnbull's Obstetrics, 2nd edition. London: Churchill Livingstone; 1995. pp. 471-88.
9. Kim JM, Park YJ. Probiotics in the prevention-treatment of postmenopausal vaginal infections: Review article. J Menopausal Med. 2017;23(3):139-45.
10. Krpina D, Raijevic-Baradic A, Palada-Kripina M. Probiotic therapy and its effects on vaginal flora. 13th World Congress in Fetal Medicine. [online] Available from https://fetalmedicine.org/abstracts/2014/abstracts/129.pdf. [Last accessed November, 2024]
11. Ledward RS, Ahmed BA. Viral infections in pregnancy. Update. 1995; 42-48.
12. Maharaj D. Puerperal pyrexia: a review. Part I. Obstet Gynecol Surv. 2007;62(6):393-9.
13. Majeroni BA, Ukkadam S. Screening and Treatment for Sexually Transmitted Infections in Pregnancy. Am Fam Physician. 2007;76(2):265-70.
14. Paladine HL, Desai UA. Vaginitis: Diagnosis-treatment. Am Fam Physician. 2018;97(5):321-9.
15. Sherrard J, Wilson J, Donders G, Mendling W, Jensen JS. 2018 European (IUSTI/WHO) International Union against sexually transmitted infections World Health Organisation (WHO) guideline on the management of vaginal discharge. Int J STD AIDS. 2018;29(13):1258-72.
16. Shlyakhov E, Segev S, Rubinstein E. Main viral diseases with in utero transmission of pathogen during pregnancy: epidemiology, pathological features and outcome. Acta Obstet Gynecol Scand. 1998;77:875-82.
17. The North American Menopause Society. Management of symptomatic vulvovaginal atrophy: 2013 position statement of The North American Menopause Society. Menopause. 2013;20(9):888-902.
18. Thulkar J, Kriplani A, Agarwal N. Utility of pH test & Whiff test in syndromic approach. Indian J Med Res. 2010;131:445-8.
19. Tomusiak A, Heczko M, Bogumił P. Antibiotic resistance of Gardnerella vaginalis. Ginekol Pol. 2011;82(12):900-4.

4

CHAPTER

Urinary Tract Infection in Pregnancy

INTRODUCTION

Urinary tract infections (UTIs) are the most common bacterial infections during pregnancy.

It can occur as:

- Asymptomatic bacteriuria
- Acute cystitis
- Acute pyelonephritis

  Asymptomatic bacteriuria: 10–13%

  Acute cystitis: 1–4%

  Acute pyelonephritis: 0.5–2%

If untreated, almost 30–40% pregnant women with asymptomatic bacteriuria will develop a symptomatic UTI.

Though incidence of bacteriuria in pregnant women is only slightly higher than nonpregnant women, the chances of progression to pyelonephritis are significantly higher, i.e., 40%.

The rate of recurrence is more in pregnancy.

PATHOPHYSIOLOGICAL CHANGES IN URINARY TRACT IN PREGNANCY

- Kidney size increases approximately by 1.5 cm.
- There is dilatation of renal calyces giving a hydronephrosis like picture. It may cause urinary stasis, thus increasing the risk of pyelonephritis.
- There is an increase in glomerular filtration rate (GFR) and renal flow rate. These changes affect the pharmacokinetics of the drugs used in treatment.
- Growing uterus compresses and laterally displaces the ureters at pelvic brim.
- Ureteral compression and effects of progesterone cause significant ureteral lengthening, dilatation, and kinking.
- These structural changes may give rise to hydroureter and sometimes obstructive nephropathy, increasing the risk of infections.
- Due to persistent pressure of gravid uterus on the bladder, there is marked thickening of bladder trigone.
- There is also increases in bladder pressure from 8 to 20 cm of water.

Due to above reasons, there is significant vesicoureteral refluxes during pregnancy, causing ascending urinary tract infections.

OTHER RISK FACTORS

- Prepregnancy history of UTI
- Lower socioeconomic status
- Sexual activity
- Older age
- Multiparity
- Anatomical urinary tract abnormalities
- Sickle cell disease
- Diabetes

ETIOLOGY

- *Escherichia coli* is most common cause of UTI, accounting for approximately 70–80%.
- *Klebsiella pneumoniae:* 5%
- *Proteus mirabilis:* 5%
- *Enterobacter* species*:* 3%
- *Group B hemolytic Streptococcus:* 2–5%
- *Coagulase-negative Staphylococcus:* 8%
- *S. aureus:* 0.9%

ASYMPTOMATIC BACTERIURIA

Significant bacteriuria in asymptomatic women is described as bacterial monoculture in the number of 10^5 colony-forming units (CFU) per mL in two consecutive mid-stream clean-catch urine specimens, according to IDSA (Infectious Diseases Society of America) criteria. Alternatively, in urine collected from a single urinary bladder catheterization, there were 10^2 CFU/mL.

American College of Obstetricians and Gynecologists as well as US Preventive Services Task Force recommend screening for bacteriuria at the first prenatal visit or at 12 weeks, whichever is earlier.

If asymptomatic bacteriuria is not treated, approximately 40% of infected women will develop symptomatic infection during pregnancy.

Untreated bacteriuria may be associated with an increased risk of preterm birth, low birth weight, and perinatal mortality.

Diagnosis

- *Urine microscopy*:
  - 10 leukocytes/HPF of the centrifuged urine sample
  - 10 leukocytes/mm^3 of uncentrifuged urine sample
- *Dipstick leukocyte esterase test:* It can be used as rapid screening test for UTI; a negative test result does not rule out UTI.

- *Urine culture:* It is collected before the first dose of antibiotic. A midstream clean-catch urine sample is collected in a sterile screw-capped container and up to a minimum volume of 10–20 mL.

Collection procedure in a catheterized patient: If the catheter is in place 14 days, replace the old catheter before collection of urine for culture. Urine samples should not be obtained from catheter bags.

Storage and transport: Transport of the specimen and plating should be done within 1 hour. If delay, the urine sample must be refrigerated at 4°C for a maximum of 6–8 hours.

Bacteriuria of 10^5 CFU/mL is associated with UTI. Any colony count is significant in symptomatic young women with pyuria. Any colony count of bacteria grown from a suprapubic aspirate is significant.

Follow-up

All pregnant women with ASB should have periodic screening after therapy, since as many as one-third of them experience a recurrent infection.

Follow-up cultures should be obtained 1–2 weeks after treatment and then repeated once a month.

ACUTE CYSTITIS

- Frequency
- Urgency
- Dysuria
- Hematuria
- Nocturia
- Suprapubic pain in the absence of systemic illness

Treatment

- Increasing oral fluid intake is frequently advocated as a first-line treatment for pregnant women with features of symptomatic urinary infection.
- Tablet nitrofurantoin SR 100 mg BD for 7 days
- Urine alkalinizing agents
- Cranberry juice also acts as urine alkalizer and is used to treat urinary infection and inhibit the symptoms.
- Fosfomycin is a new antibiotic that is taken as a single dose.
- It is a broad-spectrum antibiotic produced by certain *Streptomyces* species, and has bactericidal action.
- Administered as a single dose of 3-gram sachet
- Category B drug
- Better compliance, cost ₹ 280/sachet

Table 1 describes the various drugs that can be used for treating urinary tract infection in pregnancy.

TABLE 1: Drugs for treating UTI.

Antibiotic	*Dose*	*Duration*	*Notes*
Nitrofurantoin	100 mg orally every 12 hours	5–7 days	• Does not achieve therapeutic levels in the kidneys so should not be used if pyelonephritis is suspected • Avoid use during the first trimester and at term if other options are available
Amoxicillin	500 mg orally every 8 hours or 875 mg orally every 12 hours	5–7 days	Resistance may limit its utility among gram-negative pathogens
Amoxicillin-clavulanate	500 mg orally every 8 hours or 875 mg orally every 12 hours	5–7 days	
Cephalexin	250–500 mg orally every 6 hours	5–7 days	
Cefpodoxime	100 mg orally every 12 hours	5–7 days	
Fosfomycin	3 g orally as single dose		Does not achieve therapeutic levels in the kidneys so should not be used if pyelonephritis is suspected
Trimethoprim–sulfamethoxazole	800/160 mg (one double strength tablet) every 12 hours	3 days	Avoid during the first trimester and at term

(UTI: urinary tract infection)

ACUTE PYELONEPHRITIS

- It is the most common serious medical complication of pregnancy. Pyelonephritis was the leading cause of septic shock during pregnancy.
- In more than half of cases, pyelonephritis is unilateral and right-sided, and in a fourth of cases, it is bilateral. Fever, racking chills, and a sudden onset of pain in bilateral lumbar region, anorexia, nausea and vomiting, and tenderness elicited at costovertebral angles are the common clinical manifestations.

Complications

- Preterm labor
- Preeclampsia
- Chorioamnionitis
- Postpartum endometritis
- Low-birth weight

TABLE 2: Drugs used for treating acute pyelonephritis.

Antibiotic	*Dose, interval*
Mild-to-moderate pyelonephritis:	
Ceftriaxone	1 g every 24 hours
Cefepime	1 g every 12 hours
Aztreonam*	1 g every 8 hours
Ampicillin	1–2 g every 6 hours
plus	
Gentamicin	1.5 mg/kg every 8 hours
Severe pyelonephritis with an impaired immune system and/or incomplete urinary drainage:	
Piperacillin-tazobactam	3.375 g every 6 hours
Meropenem	1 g every 8 hours
Ertapenem	1 g every 24 hours
Doripenem	500 mg every 8 hours

* In cases of beta-lactam allergy

- Prematurity
- Developmental delay/mental retardation
- Perinatal mortality

Management

- Hospitalize patient
- Obtain urine and blood cultures
- *Blood cultures (two sets)*: Should be sent before the first dose of antibiotics if the patient is febrile, has suspected acute pyelonephritis, complicated UTI.
- Evaluate complete blood count (CBC), serum creatinine, and serum electrolytes.
- Monitor vital signs frequently, including urinary output—consider indwelling catheter.
- Establish urinary output ≥50 mL/h with intravenous crystalloid solution.
- Administer IV antimicrobial therapy **(Table 2)**
- Do a chest X-ray if there is difficulty in breathing or tachypnea.
- Repeat CBC and biochemistry studies in 48 hours.
- Change to oral antimicrobials when afebrile. Discharge when afebrile for 24 hours.
- Consider antimicrobial therapy for 10–14 days
- Repeat urine culture 1–2 weeks after antimicrobial therapy is completed.

PERSISTENT PYELONEPHRITIS

In general, intravenous hydration and antibacterial therapy are followed by a 1°F per day progressive defervescence.

Persistent infection is defined as persistent spiking fever, lack of clinical recovery after 48–72 hours, urinary tract blockage, or another consequence.

Risk Factors

- Obstruction of the urinary tract
- Ureteral or pelvicalyceal dilatation that is abnormal.
- Perinephric or intrarenal abscess
- Nephrolithiasis

Management

- Ultrasound KUB (kidney, ureter, and bladder), or intravenous pyelogram or MRI to look for persistent infection
- Cystoscopic insertion of a double-J ureteral stent to relieve obstruction
- Surgical removal of stones
- Percutaneous nephrostomy
- Duration of antibiotic treatment for complicated pyelonephritis—renal abscess, emphysematous pyelonephritis, perinephric collection, and renal obstruction—21 days

Biofilms: Uropathogenic *E. coli* (UPEC) like *E. coli* CFT073, UTI89, and 536 invades urothelial cells lining the urinary bladder which forms intracellular bacterial communities (IBCs) or biofilm.

This infection remains undetected in normal urine cultures and causes recurrence.

These culture-negative infections present as unexplained dysuria and urgency and are termed as interstitial cystitis/bladder pain syndrome.

RECURRENT URINARY TRACT INFECTION

Three or more UTIs during pregnancy are considered recurrent UTIs. Recurrent UTIs are caused by bacterial reinfection or persistence. Persistence is defined as the presence of the same germs in the urine 2 weeks following sensitivity-adjusted treatment. A reinfection is defined as a return of the same organism in >2 weeks or a sterile interim culture with a new organism.

Prevention

- Continued antibiotic prophylaxis till the end of pregnancy, in the form tablet nitrofurantoin 50–100 mg OD HS
- Intake of 150–750 mL of cranberry juice or concentrated equivalent is effective in preventing recurrent UTIs.
- Maintaining local hygiene
- Drinking at least 3–4 L of water

- Women who are sexually active, can be advised to practice postcoital voiding.

Since the urogenital flora of healthy premenopausal women is dominated by Lactobacilli, it has been suggested that restoration of the unhealthy urogenital flora from uropathogens with Lactobacilli may protect against UTI.

Promising result has been seen with intravaginal *Lactobacillus crispatus* daily for 5 days and then once weekly for 10 weeks.

No efficacy is seen with oral *Lactobacillus.*

Immunoactive Agent Prophylaxis

One of the possible pathogeneses in recurrent UTI is adaptive immune response dysfunction, especially in defects of pathogen recognition. Thus, using a vaccine to strengthen active acquired immunity against uropathogens might be a reasonable prevention of UTI recurrence. Vaginal vaccine significantly reduces the risk of recurrence of UTI. It significantly increases vaginal and urinary IgG and IgA. A recent meta-analysis published in 2013 enrolled four clinical trials of an oral vaccine (OM-89), and showed that it significantly decreased the rate of UTI recurrence. European Association of Urology Guidelines, 2015 recommend use of OM-89 for immunoprophylaxis in female patients with recurrent uncomplicated UTI.

Antimicrobial Prophylaxis

It should be used after nonantimicrobial agents have failed. Antimicrobial prophylaxis can be given consistently for long periods of time (3–6 months) or as a single postcoital dosage to prevent UTI recurrence **(Table 3)**.

Postcoital prophylaxis was found to be just as efficient as low-dose continuous antibiotic prophylaxis in preventing recurrent UTIs in a Cochrane review.

Continuous prophylaxis for 6 or 12 months reduced the rate of UTIs considerably during the prophylaxis period, but there was no difference between the two treatment groups after the prophylaxis period ended.

TABLE 3: Drugs for treating recurrent UTI.

Antimicrobial agents	*Continuous prophylaxis (daily dose) (mg)*	*Postcoital prophylaxis (one-time dose) (mg)*
Cephalexin	125–250	250
Ciprofloxacin	125	125
Nitrofurantoin	50–100	50–100
Trimethoprim/ sulfamethoxazole	40/200	40/200–80/400
Norfloxacin	200	200

(UTI: urinary tract infection)

Taking antibiotics within 2 hours of intercourse is known as postcoital prophylaxis. It takes fewer antibiotics and is associated with fewer side effects than continuous prophylaxis.

CONCLUSION

Clinical presentations include asymptomatic bacteriuria, acute cystitis, and pyelonephritis. Screening urine culture at 1st visit or at 12 weeks of pregnancy is recommended by both ACOG and RCOG for detection of asymptomatic bacteriuria. Recurrent bacteriuria in pregnancy is common and a serious cause of maternal and perinatal morbidity and mortality.

SUGGESTED READING

1. Bolton M, Horvath DJ, Li B, Cortado H, Newsom D, White P, et al. Intrauterine growth restriction is a direct consequence of localized maternal uropathogenic *Escherichia coli* cystitis. PLoS One. 2012;7:e33897.
2. Dashe JS, Bloom SL, Spong CY, Hoffman BL. Williams Obstetrics, 25th edition. New York: McGraw Hill/Medical; 2018.
3. Farkash E, Wientraub AY, Sergienko R, Wiznitzer A, Zlotnik A, Sheiner E. Acute antepartum pyelonephritis in pregnancy: a critical analysis of risk factors and outcomes. Eur J Obstet Gynecol Reprod Biol. 2012;162:24-7.
4. Gravett MG, Martin ET, Bernson JD, Khan S, Boyle DS, Lannon SM, et al. Serious and life-threatening pregnancy-related infections: opportunities to reduce the global burden. PLoS Med. 2012;9(10):e1001324.
5. Hooton TM. Urinary tract infections and asymptomatic bacteriuria in pregnancy. UpToDate.com; 2011.
6. Jolley JA, Wing DA. Pyelonephritis in pregnancy: an update on treatment options for optimal outcomes. Drugs. 2010;70:1643-55.
7. RCOG. (2012). GreenTop Guidelines No. 36: Prevention of early onset Group B *Streptococcus* infection in neonates. [online] Available from https://www.rcog.org.uk/guidance/browse-all-guidance/green-top-guidelines/prevention-of-early-onset-group-b-streptococcal-disease-green-top-guideline-no-36/. [Last accessed November, 2024]
8. Smaill FM, Vazquez JC. Antibiotics for asymptomatic bacteriuria in pregnancy. Cochrane Database Syst Rev. 2015;2019(11):CD000490.

5

CHAPTER

Puerperal Pyrexia and Sepsis

INTRODUCTION

Puerperal pyrexia: It is defined as the rise of the body temperature above 100.4°F or 38°C 24 hours apart within the first 10 days following delivery excluding the first 48 hours on two separate occasions.

The common causes of puerperal pyrexia are:

- Puerperal sepsis
- Urinary tract infection
- Caesarean scar or episiotomy site infection
- Breast abscess, mastitis
- Septic pelvic thrombophlebitis
- Respiratory infections—pneumonia

Any infection of the genital tract which is presenting as a complication of the delivery itself is called puerperal sepsis.

Most common causes include endometritis, endomyometritis, or endoparametritis.

Pelvic cellulitis is said to occur when all these present together.

DEFINITIONS

Infection: Microbial phenomenon characterized by inflammatory response to the presence of microorganisms or the invasion of normal sterile host tissue by those organisms.

Bacteremia: It is the presence of live bacteria in the bloodstream.

Septicemia: It is the presence of microorganisms or toxins in the blood.

Sepsis: Multiorgan dysfunction caused by a dysregulated host response to infection or systemic inflammation.

Maternal sepsis (World Health Organization): A life-threatening condition resulting from infection during pregnancy, childbirth, postabortion, or postpartum period causing organ dysfunction.

CLASSIFICATION FOR SEPSIS AND RELATED CONDITIONS

Systemic inflammatory response syndrome (SIRS): A host response to any of several clinical injuries, not all of which are infection (i.e., pancreatitis, trauma, severe burns).

Any two of the following need a diagnosis of SIRS:

- Temperature; 38°C or; 36°C
- Pulse rate >90/min
- Respiratory rate >20/min
- WBC count >12,000 cells/mm^3, or <4,000 cells/mm^3, >10% band forms

Severe sepsis: Sepsis with multiorgan dysfunction, hypoperfusion/ hypotension.

Hypoperfusion includes oliguria, lactic acidosis, and acute change in mental status.

Septic shock: Sepsis with hypotension (despite adequate fluid resuscitation) and hypoperfusion.

Hypotension is defined as systolic blood pressure (BP) <90 mm Hg, or when there is a reduction in systolic BP >40 mm Hg from baseline.

General variables:

- Fever (>38.3°C)
- Hypothermia (>36°C)
- Pulse rate >90/min
- Tachypnea
- Altered sensorium
- Positive fluid balance (>20 mL/kg over 24 hours)
- Hyperglycemia (plasma glucose >120 mg/dL) in the absence of diabetes

Inflammatory markers:

- Leukocytosis (WBC >12,000/μL)
- Leukopenia (WBC <4,000/μL)
- WBC normal but >10% band forms
- C-reactive protein (CRP) >2 standard deviations above normal
- Plasma procalcitonin >2 standard deviations above normal

Hemodynamic status:

- Hypotension [systolic BP >90 mm Hg, mean arterial pressure (MAP) <70, or a decrease in systolic BP more than 40 mm Hg in adults]
- SvO_2 (mixed venous oxygen saturation) >70%
- Cardiac index >3.5 L/min/m^2.

Organ dysfunction:

- Reduced partial pressure of oxygen (PaO_2) levels
- Oliguria (urine output <0.5 mL/kg/h)
- Raised creatinine >1.5 mg/dL
- Coagulation failure [international normalized ratio (INR) >1.5 or activated partial thromboplastin time (aPTT) >60 s]
- Thrombocytopenia (platelet count <100,000/μL)
- Hyperbilirubinemia (plasma total bilirubin >4 mg/dL)

PREDISPOSING FACTORS

The postpartum status of the genital tract is all together a risk factor. The placental site is an open surface after its separation covered with blood clots providing a culture media for the colonization of the bacteria. Cervicovaginal mucosa is damaged during the process of vaginal delivery. The peritoneal exposure is risk for infection during the caesarean delivery. In the lower socioeconomic strata, the maternal health status and hygiene is poor. Prelabor rupture of membranes, prolonged labor, obstructed labor, retained bits of placental products, traumatic vaginal delivery, and instrumental delivery are the other predisposing factors.

PATHOPHYSIOLOGY

The infections can be either localized or widespread to distant sites. For local infection, the primary sites are perineum, vagina, cervix, and the uterus. The damaged tissue and the blots at the perineum, vagina, and cervix promote the proliferation of the microorganisms. These local infections may spread to the uterus causing endometritis or endomyometritis.

Most commonly the decidua covering the placental site is affected.

CLINICAL FEATURES

Local infection: Red, erythematous, tender wound site, sometimes pus can be seen oozing from it. Fever, generalized weakness, and headache can be seen. High-grade fever, chills, and rigors are associated with severe infections.

Uterine infection:

- *Mild:* Fever, tachycardia, offensive lochia, and subinvolution of the uterus can be seen.
- *Severe:* High-grade fever and chills can be seen. Associated abdominal pain, dysuria, and breathlessness are present. Lochia may be scanty. Uterus tender and subinvolution can be present.

Extrauterine spread: Pelvic peritonitis is associated with high-grade fever and tachycardia.

Although other features like abdominal pain, guarding, rigidity are absent.

Tables 1 and 2 and Boxes 1 and 2 highlight the various scores which can be used for early recognition of sepsis.

If a patient screens positive for sepsis with a rapid bedside assessment, further evaluation is indicated, specifically, a careful search for infection and organ dysfunction. History, physical examination, and laboratory testing should be deployed in a focused way. Cultures should be obtained from blood and from any suspected source, but the process should not be allowed to delay initiation of antimicrobials, as delay in therapy increases mortality.

TABLE 1: Sequential organ failure assessment (SOFA) score.

System parameter	*0*	*1*	*2*	*3*	*4*
Respiratory: PaO_2/F_iO_2	• ≥ 400 mm Hg • (53.3 kPa)	• <400 mm Hg • (53.3 kPa)	• <300 mm Hg • (40 kPa)	• <200 mm Hg • (26.7 kPa) with respiratory support	• <100 mm Hg • (13.3 kPa) with respiratory support
Coagulation: Platelets (×10³/µL)	≥150	<150	<100	<50	<20
Hepatic: Bilirubin	• <1.2 mg/dL • (20 µmol/L)	• 1.2–1.9 mg/dL • (20–32 µmol/L)	• 2.0–5.9 mg/dL • (33–101 µmol/L)	• 6.0–11.9 mg/dL • (102–204 µmol/L)	• >12 mg/dL • (204 µmol/L)
Cardiovascular: MAP (mean arterial pressure)	≥70 mm Hg	<70 mm Hg	Dopamine <5 µg/kg/min, or any dose dobutamine	Dopamine 5.1–15 µg/kg/min, or epinephrine ≤0.1 µg/kg/min, or norepinephrine ≤0.1 µg/kg/min	Dopamine >15 µg/kg/min, or epinephrine >0.1 µg/kg/min, or norepinephrine >0.1 µg/kg/min
Central nervous system: Glasgow Coma Scale score	15	13–14	10–12	6–9	<6
Renal: Serum creatinine	• <1.2 mg/dL • (110 µmol/L)	• 1.2–1.9 mg/dL • (110–170 µmol/L)	• 2.0–3.4 mg/dL • (171–299 µmol/L)	• 3.5–4.9 mg/dL • (300–440 µmol/L) Or • Urine output <500 mL/day	• >5.0 mg/dL • (440 µmol/L) Or • Urine output <200 mL/day

(FiO_2: fraction of inspired oxygen; PaO_2: partial pressure of oxygen)

TABLE 2: Obstetrically modified sequential organ failure assessment (SOFA) score (omqSOFA).

	Score		
System parameter	*0*	*1*	*2*
Respiration: PaO_2/F_iO_2	≥400	300–<400	<300
Coagulation: Platelets (×10^3/μL)	≥150	100–150	<100
Liver: Bilirubin (μmol/L)	≤20	20–32	>32
Cardiovascular: MAP (mm Hg)	≥70	<70	Vasopressors required
CNS	Alert	Rousable to voice	Rousable to pain
Renal: Creatinine (μmol/L)	≤90	90–120	>120

(CNS: central nervous system; MAP: mean arterial pressure; FiO_2: fraction of inspired oxygen; PaO_2: partial pressure of oxygen)

BOX 1: Quick sequential organ failure assessment (SOFA) score (qSOFA).

Assign 1 point for each of the following. A score >1 is abnormal, and further investigation is indicated:
- Systolic blood pressure ≤100 mm Hg
- Respiratory rate ≥22/min
- Altered mental status

BOX 2: Obstetrically modified quick sequential organ failure assessment (SOFA) score (omqSOFA).

Assign 1 point for any of the following. A score >1 should prompt the clinician to consider sepsis and conduct further evaluation:
- Systolic BP <90 mm Hg
- Respiratory rate ≥25/min
- Mental status other than alert

If a patient screens positive for sepsis with a rapid bedside assessment, further evaluation is indicated, specifically, a careful search for infection and organ dysfunction.

Cultures should be obtained from blood and from any suspected source, but the process should not be allowed to delay initiation of antimicrobials, as delay in therapy increases mortality.

TREATMENT

All suspected cases of sepsis should be admitted and should be thoroughly investigated.

All other causes of fever and sepsis must be looked for.

Antibiotics should be started as soon as possible, ideally when the diagnosis of sepsis is made.

Delay in starting antibiotics increases maternal morbidity and mortality from sepsis.

Mortality from sepsis rises with each hour of delay.

Once cultures have been obtained and antibiotics started, the clinician should begin a search for a focus of infection.

Source of infection must be found promptly and all other causes should be looked for.

The choice of antibiotic depends on suspected source, likely organisms, patterns of antibiotic resistance, and the hospital's agents, but should always be broad spectrum to start.

World Health Organization recommendations for treatment of peripartum infection:

For chorioamnionitis: First-line antibiotics—ampicillin with gentamicin:

- This is very simple and effective regimen.
- It is simple, can be administered over a short period, and also it follows the principles of antibiotic use to reduce emergence of resistant strains of bacteria.

For postpartum endometritis:
"A combination of clindamycin and gentamicin is recommended."

Clindamycin may not be available in low-resource set up, so broad-spectrum penicillin can be used to cover up the infection till culture and sensitivity reports are awaited.

American College of Obstetricians and Gynecologists (ACOG) recommendations:

Primary recommendation:

- Ampicillin 2 g IV 8 hourly with *gentamicin*
  (2 mg/kg IV loading dose followed by 1.5 mg/kg q8 h, or 5 mg/kg q24 h)
- *In case of penicillin allergy:* Cefazolin 2 g IV 8 hourly with *gentamicin* (same dose)
- *In case of penicillin allergy:*
  - Clindamycin (900 mg IV 8 hourly)
    Or
  - Vancomycin (1 g IV 12 hourly) *with* gentamicin (same dose)

Other antibiotics to consider are ampicillin-sulbactam, piperacillin/tazobactam, and ertapenem. (Alternative treatments for intra-amniotic infection include cefotetan and cefoxitin, but these medications are ineffective as monotherapy.)

Fluid management in sepsis with shock: If hypotension is evident, it is the first and most important intervention. If the patient is not appropriately preloaded, he or she will have fever, venodilation, and capillary leakage.

The Surviving Sepsis Campaign (SSC) recommends a 30 mL/kg first bolus of a balanced isotonic salt solution; however, this can be too forceful during pregnancy, when colloid oncotic pressure is lower and the risk of pulmonary edema is higher.

Early intervention with a specific purpose in mind (EGDT): This necessitated the insertion of a central venous catheter, vigorous fluid resuscitation to a target central venous pressure of 8–12 mm Hg, aggressive transfusion to a hematocrit of 30%, and dobutamine as needed to achieve a goal measure of mixed venous oxygen saturation.

Vasopressors work by constricting the pathologically dilated systemic circulation seen in sepsis, allowing enough perfusion to be maintained. The SSC recommends norepinephrine as the first-line medication and suggests that mean arterial pressure (MAP) be personalized rather than set a fixed objective.

Often, clinicians must strive for a MAP of 65 mm Hg, although this may be too high for a previously healthy patient, and it is also too high during pregnancy.

Norepinephrine has been studied in human pregnancy and is used to maintain BP under regional anesthesia for caesarean.

Its safety profile is based on a dual-perfused single-cotyledon human placenta model that revealed norepinephrine did not interfere with fetal perfusion.

When there are no contraindications, norepinephrine should be administered to a septic patient.

OBSTETRIC AND PERINATAL/NEONATAL OUTCOMES

Preterm delivery is common after critical maternal illness due to sepsis.

Inflammatory mediators are released systemically which cause systemic inflammation and trigger onset of labor.

Bacteremia during pregnancy was linked to a 29% risk of preterm delivery and a 10% chance of fetal mortality in one French study, with a 40% fetal mortality rate when maternal bacteremia occurred during the second trimester. Preterm labor, premature rupture of membranes, labor dystocia, and postpartum hemorrhage are important effects.

Long-term Outcomes

There is no data available for long-term outcomes of puerperal sepsis. But incidence of morbidity and mortality is found to be raised in all the cases.

Neuropathy, myopathy, and generalized weakness are long-term consequences of ICU admitted patients.

Depression and anxiety are found to be raised among these population.

SUGGESTED READING

1. Maharaj D. Puerperal pyrexia: a review. Part I. Obstet Gynecol Surv. 2007;62(6): 393-399.
2. Ngunyi YL, Halle-Ekane G, Tendongfor N, Mbivnjo EL, Evouna Mbarga A, Nembulefack D. et al. Determinants and aetiologies of postpartum pyrexia; a retrospective analysis in a tertiary health facility in the Littoral Region of Cameroon. BMC Pregnancy Childbirth. 2020 Mar 17;20(1):167. doi: 10.1186/.

6

CHAPTER

Noninfectious Causes of Fever in Pregnancy

INTRODUCTION

It is due to chronic inflammatory conditions or autoimmune disorders like systemic lupus erythematosus. This group also comprises concept of PUO, i.e., pyrexia of unknown origin.

Pyrexia of unknown origin is defined as fever of 38.3°C or more (101°F) on several occasions, for >14 days span without any identifiable cause despite complete history, physical examination, and laboratory investigations.

Noninfectious causes for fever in pregnancy are similar to that of in nonpregnant woman.

ETIOLOGY

- *Neoplastic conditions:*
  - Lymphomas
  - Leukemia
  - Hypernephroma
- *Rheumatic and autoimmune disorders:*
  - Systemic lupus erythematosus (SLE) and rheumatoid arthritis
  - Behçet's syndrome
- *Drug induced:*
  - Sulfa drug reaction
  - Beta-lactam antibiotics
  - Antiretroviral drugs, serotonin syndrome
- *Thromboembolism:*
  - Deep venous thrombosis
  - Pulmonary embolism
- *Pulmonary causes:*
  - Acute respiratory distress syndrome (ARDS)
  - Chemical pneumonitis
- *Transfusion reactions:* Blood and blood products transfusion reaction

CLINICAL FEATURES

Table 1 highlights the differentiating characteristics seen in infectious versus noninfectious causes of fever.

TABLE 1: Differentiating features between infectious and noninfectious causes of fever.

Distinguishing infectious vs. noninfectious causes of fever:		
Signs or symptoms	***Infectious***	***Noninfectious***
Chills or rigors	+++	–
Leukocytosis*	+++	+
Pulse-temperature dissociation**	+	+++
Continuous fever***	+	+++
Hemodynamic instability and lactic acidosis	+++	–

Note: +++ (frequently occurs); + (infrequently occurs); – (does not occur)

* Acute necrotizing pancreatitis may be associated with systemic inflammatory response syndrome with leukocytosis and increased respiratory rate without evidence of an infectious process.

** Lack of increase in heart rate of 10 beats/minute per 1° of temperature increase in Celsius scale that may be present in drug-induced fever but sometimes seen in patients with infections caused by intracellular organisms (for example, pneumonia from *Legionella bacterium*).

*** Continuous fever is defined by fever that remains most of the time above 100.9°F (38.3°C).

DIAGNOSIS

- No obvious infectious cause of fever
- No history of recent hospitalization or catheterization
- History of recent travelling must be asked along with occupational history
- History of allergy or any drug intake is important

Associated symptoms will give clue regarding etiology; following associated symptoms should be looked for:

- Chills and rigors, myalgia, skin rash, joint pain, cough, dyspnea, headache, and lethargy

MANAGEMENT

Patient should be admitted and investigated carefully to rule out all possible causes of fever.

Routine ANC care is given along with fetal monitoring.

Prophylactic antibiotics are to be given and patient is monitored for pattern of fever and any other associated symptoms.

If a patient is known case of any autoimmune disease, then he/she must be evaluated for any acute exacerbation of the disease.

CONCLUSION

Pyrexia in pregnancy may not always be due to an infection. Ruling out infections, travel history, intake of any drugs, associated symptoms are crucial to point towards a noninfectious cause.

SUGGESTED READING

1. Brar R, Suri V, Suri V, Singh MP, Biswal M, Sikka P. Fever During Pregnancy: Etiology and Fetomaternal Outcomes. J Obstet Gynaecol India. 2022;72(Suppl 1):102-108.
2. Egloff C, Sibiude J, Couffignal C, Mandelbrot L, Picone O. Causes and consequences of fever during pregnancy: A retrospective study in a gynaecological emergency department. J Gynecol Obstet Hum Reprod. 2020;49(9):101899.

CHAPTER

7 Multiple Choice Questions

1. A 24-year-old G2P1L1 with 24 weeks' gestation came to OPD with complaints of per vaginal discharge. There is no history of vulval itching and its non-foul smelling. On examination, there was minimal white discharge, no vulval edema, or excoriation was seen. What will be the plan of management?

a. Antifungal pessaries

b. Kit 2 for STDs

c. Counseling of patient as it is physiological leukorrhea

d. Start her on higher antibiotics

Ans. c. Counseling of patient as it is physiological leukorrhea

2. Effects of bacterial vaginosis on pregnancy include all, *except:*

a. Preterm labor

b. Intrauterine growth restriction

c. Antepartum hemorrhage

d. Premature rupture of membranes

Ans. c. Antepartum hemorrhage

3. A 35-year-old multiparous woman came to OPD with complaint of profuse PV discharge. There was no discharge from cervix on per speculum examination. The diagnosis of bacterial vaginosis was made based on clinical findings and microscopy. All of the following will be true for this patient, *except:*

a. Presence of clue cells

b. Positive whiff test

c. Curdy white PV discharge

d. Altered vaginal pH

Ans. c. Curdy white PV discharge

4. A 29-year-old P3L3 patient who is taking ART (antiretroviral therapy) since last 10 year came to gynaecology OPD with complaint of vulval itching and PV white discharge since 1 month. On per speculum examination, curdy white discharge is seen. Most probable diagnosis is:

a. Trichomoniasis

b. Vulvovaginal moniliasis

c. Herpes simplex infection
d. Bacterial vaginosis
Ans. b. Vulvovaginal moniliasis

5. **Amsel's criteria for diagnosis of bacterial vaginosis include all, *except:***
a. Positive whiff test
b. Vaginal pH; 4.5
c. Presence of clue cells
d. Vaginal pH; 4.5
Ans. b. Vaginal pH; 4.5

6. **Which of the following organism does not directly cause vaginitis but alters vaginal flora and pH?**
a. Mobiluncus species
b. Trichomonas vaginalis
c. *Gardnerella vaginalis*
d. *Candida albicans*
Ans. c.*Gardnerella vaginalis*

7. **What is treatment of choice for mild candidial infection when it is associated with pregnancy?**
a. Topical azole therapy
b. Systemic antifungal therapy
c. Kit1 and 2 as syndromic management
d. Oral fluconazole therapy
Ans. a. Topical azole therapy

8. **Treatment of partner is essential in which of the following sexual tract infection?**
a. Bacterial vaginosis
b. Vulvovaginal candidiasis
c. Trichomoniasis
d. Moniliasis
Ans. c. Trichomoniasis

9. **The single most common cause of pyrexia of unknown origin is:**
a. *Mycobacterium tuberculosis*
b. *Salmonella typhi*
c. *Brucella* species
d. *Salmonella paratyphi A*
Ans. a. *Mycobacterium tuberculosis*

10. Pyrexia of unknown origin term is used in all of following, *except:*

a. Fever of 98°F for 1 week
b. Fever of 101°F for 2 weeks
c. No demonstrable cause of fever on evaluation
d. No recent history of travel or hospitalization

Ans. a. Fever of 98°F for 1 week

11. All of the following indicate infectious causes of fever, *except:*

a. Fever with chills
b. Fever with rash
c. Associated raised CRP
d. History of recent hospitalization

Ans. c. Associated raised CRP

12. A 24-year-old G2P1L1 with 30 weeks' gestation with known case of systemic lupus erythematosus came to OPD with history of fever since 1 day. There were no chills or rigors and no rash. She gave history of low-grade, single fever episode. What will be the line of management?

a. Evaluation to rule out other causes of fever and manage accordingly
b. Conservative treatment
c. Termination of pregnancy
d. None of these

Ans. a. Evaluation to rule out other causes of fever and manage accordingly

Index

Page numbers followed by *b* refer to box, *f* refer to figure, *fc* refer to flowchart, and *t* refer to table.

A

B

C

D

E

F

G

H

I

J

K

L

M

N

O

P

U

V

W

X